Today is the day. Make it ridiculously awesometown. Eat fruit, lots of cherries, while thinking good thoughts. ❀ Love what you do, and do it with love. Smile at strangers. Be truthful, youthful, playful, funful. Laugh at the ridiculousness of seriousness. ❀ Ride bicycles  covered in flowers. Wear colour and eat colour. ❀ Sit through the storms, for the sunshine and rainbows will follow. Eat real food. ❀ Flirt with farmers. Crunch on carrots. Labels are for tin cans. Make it from scratch. Fuel your life. Nourish your soul. Focus on the exhale. ❀ Slurp up the sunshine. ❀ Delight in the delicious. Dance like a four year-old. Offer the planet what you want the planet to offer you. Every choice counts. Optimism is most fruitful. Original over conventional. Weird over boring. Break rules. UnDiet for abundant health. Twinkle, sparkle and shine. Make Love In The Kitchen.

UnDiet

EAT YOUR WAY TO VIBRANT HEALTH

Meghan Telpner
Certified Nutritionist

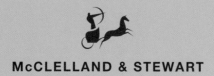

McCLELLAND & STEWART

McClelland & Stewart is a division of Random House of Canada Limited.

Published simultaneously in the United States of America by Skirt!, an imprint of Globe Pequot Press.

This publication contains the opinions and ideas of its author. It is intended to provide helpful and informative material on the subjects addressed in the publication. It is sold with the understanding that the author and publisher are not engaged in rendering medical, health, or any other kind of personal professional services. Nutritional and other needs vary depending on age, sex, and health status. If you suspect that you have a serious medical problem, the author strongly urges you to consult your medical, health or other competent professional for treatment.

Library and Archives Canada Cataloguing in Publication

Telpner, Meghan
        Undiet : eat your way to vibrant health / Meghan Telpner.
Includes index.
ISBN 978-0-7710-8411-9
        1. Telpner, Meghan – Health. 2. Self-care, Health. 3. Healing. I. Title.

RA776.95.T42 2012   613   C2012-903511-4

All photos, with the exceptions below, by Catherine Farquharson.
Image on page 5 courtesy of Kristin Rugg Dovbniak; image on page 64 courtesy of Bryan Goman; personal photos by Meghan Telpner Inc.; chapter opener illustration by Dorothy McMillan
Typeset in Perpetua
Printed and bound in China

McClelland & Stewart,
a division of Random House of Canada Limited
One Toronto Street
Toronto, Ontario
M5C 2V6
www.mcclelland.com

1   2   3   4   5   17   16   15   14   13

For my Baba Rose and Grandpa Gene.
You would have been the proudest of all.

Courage and cheerfulness will not only carry you over the rough places
in life, but will enable you to bring comfort and help to the weak-hearted
and will console you in the sad hours.

— SIR WILLIAM OSLER

A wise man should consider that health is the greatest of human blessings,
and learn how by his own thought to derive benefit from his illnesses.

— HIPPOCRATES

CONTENTS

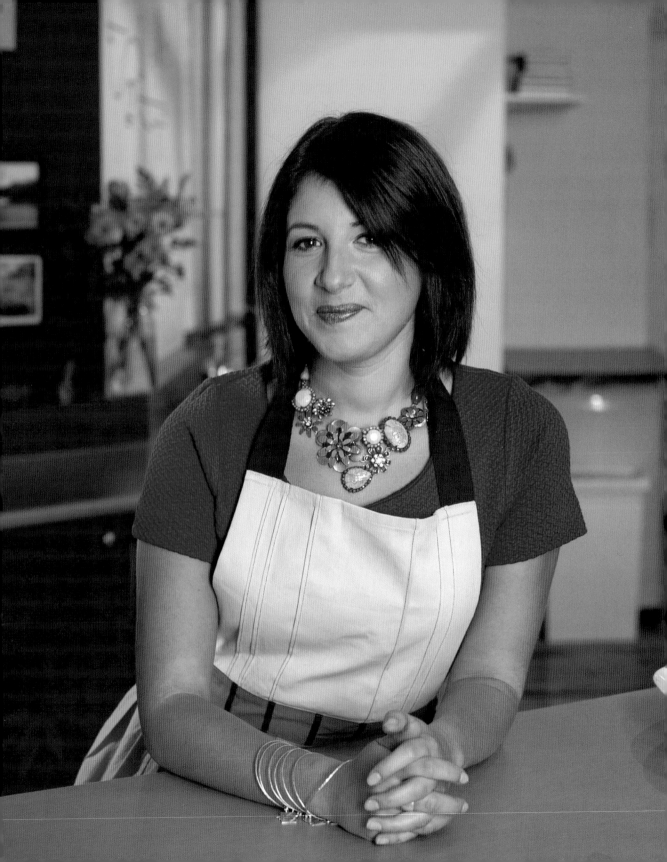

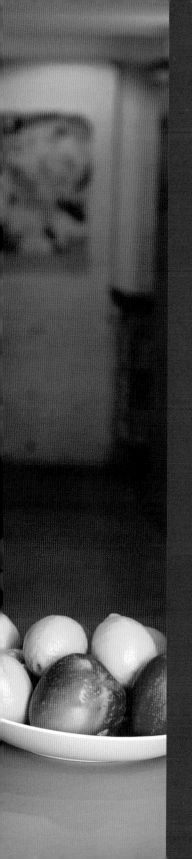

Nutritionista at Your Service

Greetings, salutations, and a back-handspring, triple-flip welcome to the land of UnDieted love, super fun, and a dash or two of awesometown. Thank you kindly for choosing me to assist you on this adventure we are about to embark upon together.

I'll bet you're a little curious about how I came to be doing this kind of cheerleading for abundant, vibrant living. I am, by training, a certified nutritionist. I went to school, studied, and learned a whole lot to earn the honor of wearing that title – but *nutritionista* sounds more fun. As a nutritionista, my mission is to get you looking and feeling amazing, without making you weigh your food, portion out three almonds for a snack, or employ a calculator to count the calories and ounces of this or that. My entire philosophy around health, and the roundabout path that took me from being a fashion school grad to singing and dancing to the tune of healthy living, evolved by way of my own severe health challenges.

Despite how sweetly this profession fits, I hardly came by it naturally — or should I say "organically"? I didn't grow up eating sprouts and had never heard of sauerkraut before, let alone considered making my own. My family ate pretty well, but I was more familiar with macaroni-and-cheese from a box, white-bread sandwiches, and rolled up fruit snacks than I was with brown rice, kale, or a smoothie. Up until my late twenties, I was not a person who loved being in my kitchen, had an interest in alternative medicine, or even gave much thought to my health. A nutritionist was certainly not what I had aspired to be.

The roundabout path to becoming a nutritionist included a degree in fashion, travels through rural Africa, a career in advertising, and exploding intestines. I didn't get into nutrition and health until I had to; I didn't learn to make brown rice, kale, and smoothies (often with kale in them) until I had exhausted all other avenues. Most of us come by natural health through desperation and my story is no different. Some of the information being shared in these colorful pages is what I learned through my extensive formal education earning my nutritionist certification, as well as through intensive post-graduate study. Most of it though, the really great nuggets that set *UnDiet* apart from every other health, diet, and lifestyle guide, are the *Why didn't I ever think of that?, That's such a great idea!* and *I have to give this a try!* juicy "a-ha" bits of info I have learned through everyday practice as I strive to maintain optimal health, and also in my work motivating, challenging, and hopefully inspiring others to do the same.

Some of my own transitions were very abrupt — illness often forces us to do things we might never have previously considered. Most of the changes however have been gradual, simply learning as I live. The way I see it, the UnDiet lifestyle is a bit like yoga — it is a practice. All we can do is just keep practicing, hopefully getting a little better every day, as we continue to learn new things and incorporate a little more into our lives.

I'll be totally honest here: every morning I am mildly astounded when I juice my greens, pack up my lunch, and ride my bike over to the Meghan Telpner Inc. headquarters, that my personal desire to feel great has fueled more than a journey toward my own personal health. I never expected that I would become a teacher of abundant living for others or that I'd continue learning right alongside my students, and will forever be teaching at the edge of my own knowledge. There is no division between the work that I do and the life that I live. I practice what I preach to the very best of my abilities.

This health thing is ongoing and will always be changing to suit our needs. My approach is to make healthy living as fun as possible: take what you can, leave what you're not ready for, and maybe you'll come back later and give it a try.

RECIPES MADE (EASILY) WITH LOVE
As much as I like to pretend I've got my chef whites on when I'm in my kitchen, **I am not a trained chef**. I taught myself to cook by learning about the powerful healing benefits of key foods, and then figuring out fun ways to make them. While the main rule was that everything had to be health-promoting, what was more important was that everything also be delicious and nice to look at. Therefore, my recipes have become known for three important things: their yumminess, their **prettiness**, and their ease. That's what I have here for you, in *UnDiet* – yummy, pretty, and easy recipes. And, here's an added bonus: they are all **gluten-free**, dairy-free, and vegetarian (always with vegan options), with a concentration on package-free, from-scratch cooking. I haven't a clue what the calorie counts are on these recipes and quite frankly, it doesn't matter (you're about to understand why!). Be sure to check them out; they just might change the game for you!

NICE PICTURES!
Why, thank you! They are nice, aren't they? Many of the photos throughout this book are my own personal shots from my own personal life. If you see a picture and wonder, *What is going on here? Where is she? Who is she with? What is she doing?* just hop over to http://bit.ly/UnDiet for the story behind it and others in this book.

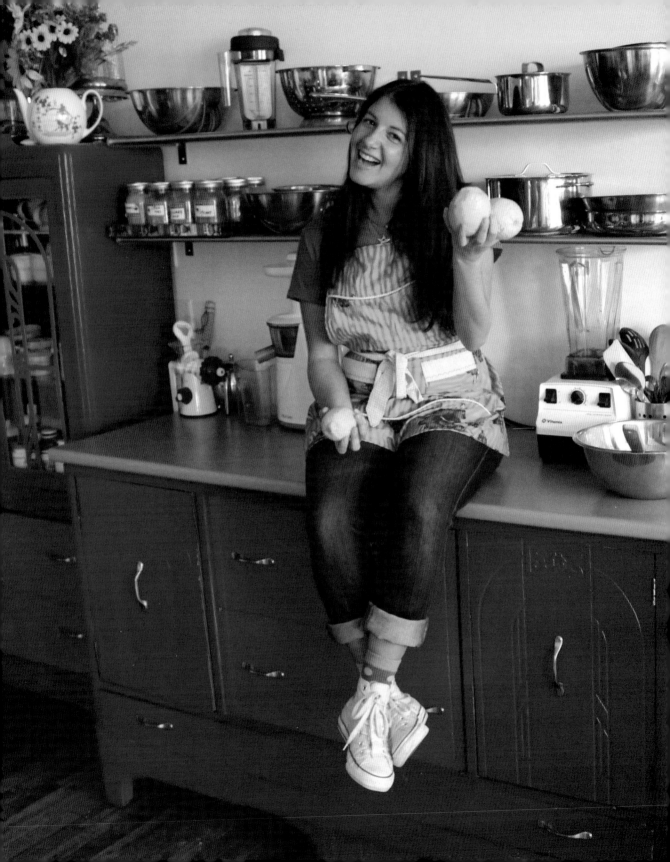

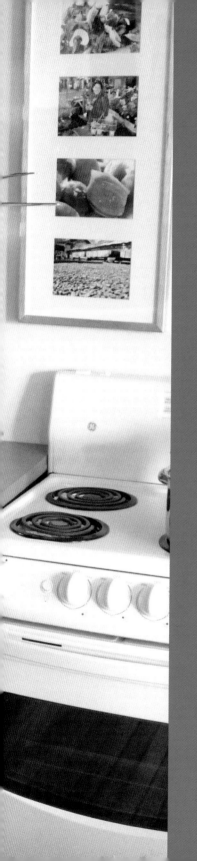

CHAPTER 1

Eat Your Way to Vibrant Health

FROM FASHIONISTA TO NUTRITIONISTA

When we have no choice but to face our greatest fears, we have a choice to make: succumb to what we're being told, or dig way deep down to find the super-hero bravery that allows us to seek alternatives. I opted for the latter and – wowza! – did that take me on a journey I hadn't signed up for. This, my sweet and lovely health adventurer, is how I became a nutritionista.

My health challenges began in August of 2003 when, after graduating with first-class honors and a Bachelor of Applied Arts in fashion, I decided to head to Africa alone. I know it doesn't make a whole lot of sense: a little five-foot-nothing fashionista, vying for a career in the world of glam, seeking adventure in rural Mozambique and Swaziland with only a backpack and a slew of vaccination certificates stuffed into her passport. So it was, though.

In late August, a week after receiving my vaccination cocktail for the trip, I fell ill. I had flu-like symptoms, a fever, chills, and was doubled over with severe stomach pains. As I boarded the plane for Africa, I still had not fully recovered. By the time I returned home ten weeks later, in mid-December 2003, things had gotten worse, so I began my tour of physicians, specialists, holistic practitioners, and therapists to find out what was going on.

March of 2004 rolled around and I landed a job with an ad agency. As I began the climb up the corporate ladder from my lowly bottom-rung position, I struggled with my health. No one could tell me what was wrong. My tests kept showing up fine, but my symptoms (stomach pain, cramping, gurgling, intermittent diarrhea with constipation, resulting in sleep deprivation) got worse, as my worries grew.

I am pretty sure we all have those experiences in our lives, when we look back and ask ourselves, quite seriously, *What was I thinking?* For some time following my African adventure, this question somersaulted in my head while it felt as if another creature did cartwheels in my tummy.

Despite my doctors' conviction that stress was more of a culprit than my diet, and that lifestyle and hormones were perhaps to blame, I couldn't get past the fact that the day before my vaccinations I had been fine and one week later, everything began to fall apart. No one seemed able to work out what could make it all stop; no one could help me get well.

As my symptoms progressed, my diet became more limited. I developed this intense fear of eating; never knowing whether what I ate was going to make me feel amazing, or take my insides on a Tilt-A-Whirl. I followed what my doctors, naturopaths, and friends told me to try but continued getting worse.

Three years and nineteen doctors later, in August of 2006, I was diagnosed first with ulcerative colitis and later with Crohn's Disease, an autoimmune, inflammatory bowel disease that can affect any part of the digestive tract from the mouth to the exit point. My gastroenterologist informed me of treatment options that were scarier than the disease itself. Medications were the only immediate option to try and manage the increasingly severe symptoms, followed by the possibility of surgery if the disease progressed. The idea of having my guts sliced with a scalpel to remove a portion of an organ that, even with my limited understanding of anatomy, I imagined had been put there for good reason, was unthinkable. I was being offered a lifetime of medications, emergency rooms, surgeries, and my greatest fear of all — a colostomy bag. I didn't want my intestines replaced by a bag, worn outside my body, to collect my poop. This option was *not* an option. I was terrified.

The vision I had of what my future would be — cute boyfriend, career in advertising, plenty of travel — was suddenly up for grabs. The only question I could ask was *How do I make this disease go away?* My doctor explained that I couldn't. There was no cure. At the age of twenty-six, I was given little hope of ever regaining perfect health. My doctor explained, "You're young, have fun, drink your milkshakes, eat your cheeseburgers. Nothing you eat is going to affect the prognosis of your disease. You're going to have to learn to live with it."

I was no expert on human biology, but I began to think that a disease of the digestive tract must be affected by what passes through it. Since surgery and medication are not cures, I was willing to take my chances on some natural remedies, which would at least help me get stronger should I require medication and surgical intervention — and maybe even actually help me heal.

I had spent the three years since first getting sick doing what I had been told, following rules and guidelines and dietary advice. It hadn't worked. It became clear that I had to be brave enough to start making some choices for myself. If what I was currently doing wasn't working, I could either give up and give in, or take the tougher route — take ownership and responsibility for my health. It was time to start breaking the rules. It was time to UnDiet.

I spent hours on the Internet: reading, writing to people, and asking questions. I disregarded a lot and remembered the bits that made sense to me — much of which contradicted what my doctors had told me.

Health is our natural birthright. If we give our body what it needs to heal, and let our mind rest, the body will take care of itself. I felt as if I'd found a secret exit out of this downward spiral and chose to dive through with streamers flying and pom-poms pomming. I made the decision, with absolute conviction, that I was going to do a little dance, make a little love in the kitchen, and get myself well by breaking the rules of convention. I traded in my working-girl outfits for flip-flops, a yoga mat, and a bicycle with a basket I decorated with flowers. I was too sick to work regular hours and so I took a

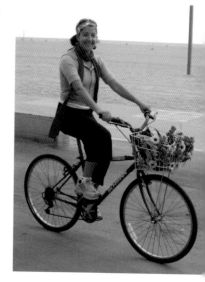

leave of absence to take on my new full-time job: healing. I wasn't searching for a magic cure. My goal was to heal the disease and make it go away.

I decided that in order for this to work, healing would have to be the most fun I'd ever had in my whole life, because the alternative, getting worse, was unthinkable. Six days a week for three months, I went for acupuncture. Acupuncture helped me to relax, first and foremost. It got my energy, or *Chi*, flowing. It accelerated the physical healing of the lesions in my intestines, strengthened my immune system, and supported my nervous system. A body cannot heal when it is in a stressed or anxious state; both the mind and the body have to be united in this commitment. With my remaining free time, I did loads of reading on food, cooking, and healing, and I discovered how to flirt with farmers to get the best bunches of kale and crispiest apples at the market. I learned to sit still in silence while simultaneously taking deep breaths into my belly (they call this meditating, you know). I gave up my television, my gym membership, and my hot-to-trot English boyfriend. Nothing was going to distract me from the goal; nothing was more important to me than this.

I vowed to do six things every day:

* Meditate twice.
* Take a morning walk.
* Nap if I was tired.
* Go to yoga, even if all I did was lie down for the whole class.
* Eat food prepared completely from scratch and have fun doing it.
* Do absolutely nothing if that's what I wanted to do.

The goal was to be easy on myself, not force anything, but simply to undo all that I had done that had contributed to this disease. I did as much of this as I could with a laugh and a smile, even if I didn't much feel like doing either.

I was excited by what I was learning, how I was feeling, and who I was meeting. My mom told me I was getting my Ph.D. in life. All I knew was that simplifying everything, reducing my need for material goods, and just being easier on myself, felt like a giant exhale after holding my breath all my life.

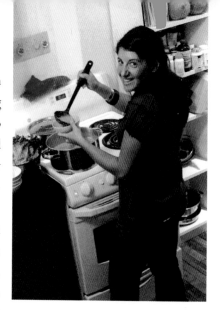

Most profound, however, was my discovery of that room in my house called the *kitchen*. I knew that if I was really going to get well and healthy, I had to learn to cook. I would have to ignore the false and misleading "healthwashing" claims splashed across packaged foods. I would need to UnDiet my diet by going against conventional dietary recommendations and mass-produced processed food.

As I began to heal and could tolerate more foods, I began experimenting. I would start with a whole food, eat it plain Jane by itself, then slowly build on it, learning about herbs and spices, flours, oils, and vegetables, until I created recipes. Cooking became the highlight of my day. As I healed, I expanded my diet with only one rule governing my choices: the ingredients had to be whole. All the processing had to happen in my kitchen so no vital parts of the food would be left out, and no poison-like additives or preservatives would be added in.

get the stories
behind the photos
http://bit.ly/UnDiet

The UnDiet began to rule my world and the result was that after one month, I was 100 percent symptom-free from a disease believed to have no cure. I did this by breaking the rules, cleansing out the bad stuff, making space for the good, living wholly and fully with joy and pleasure. The outcome was beautiful, abundant health, and I knew that this way of living and eating couldn't end once I was feeling better. My previous lifestyle had contributed to my ill health and I did not want to repeat it. I was wise enough to know that this wasn't a crash diet and that I could not resume past habits once I felt better. This was now simply my way of living; my lifestyle of choice.

Going back to advertising was not an option; the stress and long hours clearly hadn't worked. So I did something I was pretty sure I would never do: I went back to school and earned my certification as a nutritionist. From the moment I started down this path, I worked my booty off to learn as much as I could, break rules every day, and question conventional paradigms. I was determined to continue to UnDiet my life along a path of total health.

The result of this journey is that I have become the person that I needed to meet all those years ago. Of course, given my nature, had I met me nine years ago, there is no way I would have listened. These were lessons I had to learn myself.

STRATEGIES TO HELP YOU BE THE SUPPORT
BY MEGHAN'S MOM, PATSY TELPNER

Seeing Meghan go through what she did, I knew she was going to have to take this on herself. The toughest part was watching her struggle to find the right path. What she has achieved with her health is inspiration for us all. No matter who in your life is dealing with a challenge, there are some strategies that can promote health for everyone involved.

❀ **Be Informed:** The best thing you can do, if you're feeling helpless, is to get informed. It will help you advocate, when needed, for the person suffering and often for your own peace of mind. You will be empowered with the knowledge you need to ask the right questions and understand the answers.

❀ **Be There:** Be okay with knowing your help may not be wanted all the time. The person going through the crisis is having a tough time too; let them go through it knowing you are there, without judgment, if they need you.

❀ **Be Careful:** There is nothing worse than being pestered with everyone else's opinions. The recipient might be feeling overwhelmed, scared, or simply not interested. That is his or her choice.

❀ **Be Quiet:** Easier said than done, but learn to do it. Anyone on a path to health has to find his or her own way. Nagging and pestering will likely lead to greater rebellion.

❀ **Be Okay:** Helping someone else heal can be tough on you. They likely won't do what you would do in that situation, but you can't control that. You have to mind your own stress and worry and learn and develop the tools you need to cope.

Patsy Telpner is Meghan's momma and she gives the best advice. Acting as Meghan's personal advisor on all matters for the better part her whole life, this woman knows what she's talking about.

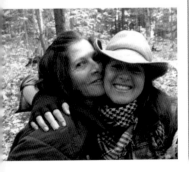

LESSONS OF UNDIETING

Healing from Crohn's taught me a thing or ten. As with all truly horrific, nightmarish events that we have in our lives, we can decide to make it the worst thing to ever happen to us, or the very best. What I learned with everything I went through is that there is really no point in dwelling on the negatives. We cannot change what happens to us, my dear sweet coconut sugar, but we can totally change how we respond, react, process, and move forward.

It was with this state of mind that I embraced the change that needed to come into my life. And it wasn't always a bicycle ride along the beach. There were days, and times, and changes that were really, really hard. There were days when I would call my mom in tears, having what she described as a meltdown. There were days when I doubted what I was doing and feared that maybe there was good reason for convention; maybe there was a reason we all followed a similar diet and abided by the same rules. I feared that I would look foolish, that the plan would backfire, that I would get more sick, and that my doctor and the eighteen before him would collectively look down their noses at me smugly and grin with a big giant "I told you so," as their scalpels glimmered under the surgical lights, hovering just above my intestines.

And when I had enough of playing the woe-is-me game, I would get on my bike, go for a ride, or lie down, take some deep breaths, and accept that right now, in this very moment, I am perfectly okay.

The more I began to accept that the present moment was the only truth I could rely on or trust, it became easier to follow my instincts, to continue to undo old ways of living and thinking. I learned lessons that I believe we will all learn when we follow the path we create for ourselves, questioning convention and ultimately UnDieting our way to a new and elevated way of living.

"Each experience in your life was absolutely necessary
in order to have gotten you to the next place,
and the next place, up to this very moment."
– Dr. Wayne Dyer

TEN THINGS YOU'LL LEARN UNDIETING TO VIBRANT HEALTH

1

How to Cook ... Really Well. We think cooking is this complicated process that requires a weird-looking white hat, a set of gabillion-dollar knives, and words like *flambé*, *al dente*, and *bouquet garni*. What I learned and what you will too is that amazingly delicious cooking is easy. Super easy. It is not about fancy-pants techniques, but starting out with the freshest of fresh ingredients, and doing as little to them as possible. When we take great-quality ingredients, the way we prepare them or combine them to bring out their most amazing flavor also often ends up being the healthiest way to consume them.

You don't have to be a chef to make the best tasting food; it's simply about being open to trying new tastes, foods, and textures, and exploring that room in the house called *the kitchen*. In fact, you will discover how to make sweet, sweet love in the kitchen. I promise two things:

❉ You will not be spending every waking moment in the kitchen.
❉ You may wish you could spend every waking moment in the kitchen.

2

Take Other People's Opinions with a Grain of Salt. Sometimes we have to listen to what other people have to say. Other times we can add their opinion to the equation, as part of the decision-making process. And then there are the times when someone's opinion so firmly disagrees with every part of us, especially that little inkling in the belly often referred to as intuition or instinct, that it is in our best interest to totally and completely ignore it. I received the opinion that I had an incurable disease and nothing I ate or did regarding my diet or lifestyle would have an effect. I chose to trust my own opinion that this was not true. That has made all the difference.

Part of the UnDiet is creating our own rules. I may suggest something to you, and someone else might tell you something different. I am not in your body or your mind. I don't know how you feel. Only you do. This means that sometimes, you are just going to have to make up your own mind based mostly on your own opinions. With that being said, when I suggest, *Hey Sunshine, lay off the sugar, it's adding junk to your trunk and turning you into a total cranky-pants*, that may not be the best time to totally disregard my opinion because your own opinion is that *a little is okay*, or *I hate when she says that because all I want right now is a giant ice cream sundae to drown out the feeling that I might really need a hug right now.*

Breaking the rules to UnDiet means knowing when you really do have to play by the broken rules, and not let your own thoughts, fears, boundaries, or mind games get in the way of über-powered UnDiet success.

You picking up what I'm putting down here? Taking another's opinion with a grain of salt is one thing, ignoring it because it seems hard, or painful, or challenging, or transitional, or uncomfortable is a total cop-out.

The Writing Is Always on the Wall. The message we are supposed to heed, for the most part, is so flipping clear that we fail to notice it. The old saying hindsight is twenty-twenty is an annoying truth. It is so easy to see afterward what we were supposed to see or do, but often in the moment, our heads are buried so deep analyzing the past and fretting about the future that we don't notice the present until we are literally knocked over. We fail to look up until we are brought to our knees.

3

In those moments, when we realize that we failed to notice the neon-sign writing flashing across the wall of our life (often in the form of physical pain, recurring illness, recurring overly dramatic-bawl-your-eyes-out relationships, or poor career moves), we have the opportunity to wake up. We have to learn to read the writing on that wall, with clean spectacles, and free of the fear that kept our heads down in the first place, for if we don't, the messages will come back again and again, and likely more painful and aggressive each time.

This is one of the greatest times to start UnDieting your life to a higher place. There is no need to give this power away to a leader, a guru, a doctor, or your mother/lover/brother/sister/best friend. Trying to follow what someone else says or dictates may seem like the easy way, as it frees us from taking responsibility. And it may just

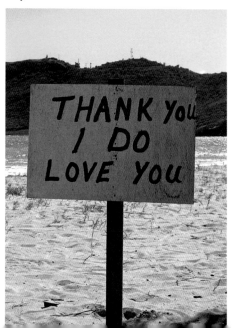

be the easy way . . . for a time. But it won't work long term. This is the time to stop looking for answers to healing outside ourselves. It is time to focus on the exhale, look within, and, goodness me almighty, we will find the answers there. We just have to be brave enough to stop and take a look at what's really going on – and to listen.

4 **Yoga Is More than Twisting Yourself into a Pretzel.** Remember just a flash ago where I said we have to be brave enough to stop for a moment and see what's up in our heart and head and body? This is where yoga comes in. And before you let that soundtrack play in your head that declares your body not flexible enough to do yoga, that, my lovers, is what we call your ego mixed up with the covers of *Yoga Journal* magazine. Yoga is about stopping, breathing, and going within. A walk can be yoga if you want it to be. So can golfing. There is no need to stretch your knee behind your head to gain perspective and calm.

Here's the thing. High-intensity workouts allow you to stay on the outside of yourself. You get to stand in front of a mirror where one of two things will happen. You may look at yourself and think, *My oh my, I am hot stuff today. Check out my biceps? Look at my bum lifted firmly off the backs of my legs.* Or you might be the type to think, *Seriously! Why did I eat that last night? I'll never get a date as long as I look like this. No wonder I can't get that promotion. My flibbidy-flabby thighs are getting in the way of professional success.* No matter what story plays in your head, neither one is getting you to go inside. And for the record, your thighs are not the reason why you didn't get the promotion.

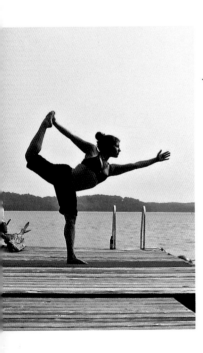

Yoga forces us to move slowly, and focusing only on the breath forces us to ask the really big questions. For this reason, yoga is a gazillion times harder than climbing a stair-climber and doing crunches until you want to puke. Yoga makes you actually look at yourself from the inside; it holds up a mirror and forces us to pay attention. We cannot heal what we don't touch and if we don't deal with our own stuff, the shadow keeps coming out. The deeper your practice becomes, the more you are asking yourself to take ownership over your life.

As we check our calorie-counting and heart-rate monitors at the UnDiet door, we also stop letting our limited beliefs keep us from seeing the world in the most real way.

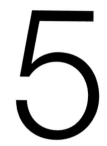

Wait Out the Storms, and Sunshine and Rainbows Will Appear – If You're Looking. I'll be the first to admit that sometimes life just plain old bites the big one. Things get tough and sticky, icky, and prickly. Shifting any belief system such as going from a conventional diet to the awesome-town UnDiet way of living might result in a few storm clouds. People will ask you questions, think you're a nutter, and send you studies that don't make a whole lot of sense but disagree with what you've decided to do for yourself. Transitioning away from foods you've been hooked on or putting an end to staying up until 1:00 a.m. looking at friends' pictures on Facebook might have some of the uncomfortable feelings of withdrawal that come from an end to any addiction.

And then sometimes events happen that look as though they may derail any hope for the goodness we are working on building. But see, that's okay. Life can be messy and cloudy sometimes. The secret is to not hold on to the rainy days and expect that every morning we will wake up to another dark and grey rainstorm of a day. There is always a silver lining, that sweet rainbow when the clouds clear. The challenge is that if we don't look for it, we will never see it.

What it all comes down to here is that we can't control much in our life. What we can control, or at least work on, is how we respond and react in any given situation. The UnDiet is a process of undoing many bad habits, to make space for the good, the rainbows. It's a process of building up enough strength to change our perspective of an experience, our lifestyle, or our ambitions and goals for our life, without doing away with the negative or wishing for it to have passed us by. The stormy days, weeks, or years that may bring us down will provide the answers that will ultimately raise us up to greater heights.

At the end of the day, sometimes life does suck monkey balls. That just means we're going to have to learn to love monkeys.

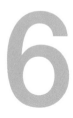

A Cute Outfit Doesn't Mean Much When You Feel Like Total Crappola. This lesson, which we all learn at one time or another, goes back to the whole point about working out the bum cheeks. See, the exercised bum will look great in a new pair of hipster jeans, but what happens when we feel too unwell to go out and show off our great ass? The look-at-my-great-ass hipster jeans won't be cheering us up as they hang in our closet.

The oddest thing for me, when I was sick and became a skinny minny, was that so many people were telling me how great I looked. As I got healthier and gained the weight back, and kept being told how "healthy" I looked, I thought this was a nice word for "fat." What I had to accept was the simple notion that I'd rather have a full head of curly hair, nails that would grow, a body that let me eat and digest my food, a mind that could let me sleep at night, and carry a little more roundness in my bootylicious behind than be sick.

It takes time to understand that great health means so much more than cute shoes and manicured nails. When we feel strong, well, and balanced on the inside, it radiates through every pore of our being. Internal mind and body health precedes all external surface beauty.

When we feel amazing on the inside, we can wear a paper bag and be the belle of the ball. For many, some of the most challenging transitions in the UnDiet will be those that affect outward appearance, but have trust and faith; you will be sending thank-you notes my way in the end. No Fendi handbag or Hermes scarf will make your day when you are bawling your eyes out with PMS, bedridden with a migraine, or trapped in the loo with an irritable bowel.

7 Always, Always, Always Trust Your Intuition. In the time I was going from doctor to doctor, I was also going from job to job. I would be offered a new position and write up a pro-and-con list of what was great and what was not so great. Things that fell on the pro side were often *cute guy at desk near boardroom, office has windows that open,* and *office closes between Christmas and New Year's.* Eight jobs in three years should have been a sign that I was doing the wrong thing. The truth is that we always inherently know the right thing to do.

We've all had those icky sticky relationships with the high highs and low lows that for some reason keep us hooked, right? For me, I knew in my heart it was totally not the right thing and I would meditate on it, asking myself *What should I do?* I would expect this subtle message, but what I always got was a blasting *GET OUT GET OUT GET OUT!*

The problem I had with my jobs and with the dirtbag boyfriends was never that I didn't know the right thing to do, but that I didn't want to listen.

My oldest friend Jay has a saying, *When there's doubt, there's no doubt*. Let that sink in for a moment. Basically, we always know what's right, right?

As we move through the following chapters, you will likely have an easy time with some of the switcheroos and more of a challenge with others. A challenge, having to put in some extra effort, is not a doubt. As you continue to UnDiet your life, much of what is here will make absolute perfect sense because it is fully in line with what your intuition has been telling you all along.

Intuition never lies, we just have to get out of our heads long enough to tune into that inkling of a feeling that will always guide us in the right way. And if you can't hear it, it could mean that your life is too noisy. Be still a little bit every day and you will start to hear the voice, and over time you will learn to listen. And over even more time, you will learn to trust that it is *always* right.

You Are About to Be an Inspiration (Even Though You Likely Already Are). Being an inspiration is very simple. Doing something in our lives that other people deem impossible in theirs makes us inspiring. Giving up sugar can be just as inspiring as climbing a mountain. If both are done with grace, commitment, and determination, then both are inspiring. And I bet you could find someone who has climbed to the highest peak of the highest mountain who wouldn't dare brave a sugar detox.

Being an inspiration is not about the things we practice but the way we practice them. If we are able to do what we do, no matter what that is, with true love and true integrity, then my fair inspirer, you are, no doubt, a total and complete inspiration.

Leaping into the UnDiet with a skip in your step and a smile on your face – and doing your very best to keep it there through each tip, suggestion, transition, and cleanse-out – will make you a super inspiration!

By the time you are done, you will feel so fantabulous and so inspired by yourself, that you'll likely already be on to your next great inspiring endeavor. That's just how inspiration works. It's like going down a steep hill on roller skates without learning to use the brakes – sometimes it's a little scary, but the wind in your face and the views along the way keep you moving along and the next thing you know you're doing turns and back flips in the air. Roller skating is fun.

9

Fighting for Something to Be Different Doesn't Help It to Heal.
Is it too early in the UnDieting game to bring up a touchy issue? A key to UnDieting is breaking the rules and one such rule is that we have to fight to achieve. That's just silly. Things don't have to be hard to be right. In fact, the easiest solution is usually right in front of us. My meditation teacher told me the story of the brick wall. The short version is simply that if we can take a break from tearing down the brick wall and step back for a moment we're likely to find the open door right there beside us, and it has been there all along.

Canada spends more than $450 million a year on cancer-related research, with only 2 percent allocated to prevention,[1] and the United States spends $5 billion per year fighting for a cure.[2] Is it possible they may be looking for it in the wrong place? Few people take the time to look down into their shopping carts or in their shower to see the scary ingredients they consume and use daily that have been linked to cancer, let alone acknowledge lifestyle habits or even their own stressful thoughts as potential contributors. Fighting for something rarely gets us the outcome we desire. In relationships, fighting for the one you love usually freaks him or her out and leaves you all by your lonesome. Fighting to get that raise or promotion will earn you enemies and resentments. Fighting the bulge will make you pack it on, and fighting for peace . . . well, we know how that one goes.

How do we heal? Well, what do you do when you get a paper cut? Do you burn all the paper and cut off your fingers? No. We need paper. And fingers. You let it be, maybe put an agent on it to help it heal, cover it with a bandage to protect it, and let the body do what it does really well when we get out of the way – it heals.

With every TV commercial and "reality" makeover show, we have come to crave instant results from dramatic interventions. We have put our aggressive nature into trying to change what is, which only seems to create more resistance. What if, instead, we look at how we can *work with* what is, instead of fighting against it? What if we resolve our health challenges by working with them, by offering the body, mind, and our lives what we need to heal, repair, and thrive long term, instead of constantly fighting against it with aggressive, ineffective, short-term interventions?

Happily Create Instead of Creating to Be Happy. Here is the big old granddaddy of lessons. We think that if we work now, even if we hate it, that the benefits or payoff will bring happiness to the future version of ourselves. Ever tried to starve yourself on a calorie-restricted diet? What about slugging away at a job you hate, counting down the days to the weekend or to your next holiday, thinking that you have to do this now, in order to gain the rewards of happiness later?

Take a moment, if you would, and think back one year, five years, maybe ten years. Think about what you were doing, maybe who you were doing, and what seemed the most important thing in your life. Think about what you were working so hard to get. Did you get it? Is what you were struggling to get through then bringing you happiness now? Is it even what you want now?

Seems to me that being miserable now, thinking that misery will bring us some great reward of happiness in the near or distant future, is a waste of precious time. That happy place in the distant future will always remain just out of reach. Why take on misery now in order to achieve something that is only serving to satisfy and bring joy to a future version of ourselves?

We will find ourselves pretty disappointed for a good portion of our lives. Things can change in an instant, with a diagnosis, a disaster, or even minor missteps in the day. The greatest gift we can offer ourselves is to wake up happy, excited about the day ahead, and go to bed pleased with the job that we did, accepting that the process itself is the outcome, and that we did our very best at every given moment.

QUESTIONING THE PARADIGMS

Questioning paradigms is the quickest way to become the outcast at a dinner party. I'm serious. It's nice to sit around with our friends and talk about Hollywood movies, great new shops and restaurants, our recent holiday in Puerto Vallarta, and our adventures in the housing market.

But what happens when you announce that you're replacing your microwave with a juicer? Giving up coffee? Quitting your job, abandoning the security of the cubicle, to start that stationery business you've always dreamed of? What if you decide to pull your kids from school and travel around the world for a couple years? What if you decide to boycott the aisles of the supermarket and eat solely from the perimeter? What if you tell your friends you're going to go off your anti-anxiety medications and instead try a month-long meditation retreat? What if you are diagnosed with an incurable disease and instead of getting your intestines cut out, you decide to get acupuncture and drink shots of wheatgrass and herbal teas?

What if you asked those same friends, at that same dinner party, what medications they are currently on and what they would be willing to do to stop taking them? Would they replace their microwave with a juicer? Would they give up coffee? They'd probably look at you like you've lost your marbles.

It is strange to me that people refer to someone as "the healthy one in the family," or describe the taste of food as "healthy," as if that were a bad thing. Wouldn't you rather be described as the healthy one than the sick one? Wouldn't you rather eat something that tastes healthy than something that tastes like it might cause you to have a quadruple bypass? Strangely, for most people, they'll take the bypass. Play now, pay later.

When we start to ask these questions, we start to question the paradigms of what is considered normal and to do things that are a little different, or what some may call abnormal. I prefer to call it being conscious. What I have come to discover is that the people who live on the periphery, with one foot in the "normal" world and the rest in their own world, have the ability to do things differently, be okay with it, be respected for it, and perhaps inspire new directions for others.

When my father was diagnosed with cancer in 2010 and he opted to break the rules right along with me and employ a veg-loving diet that included juicing and therapeutic supplements, people thought he was playing a dangerous game. The common perception is that high doses of nutrition is more terrifying than getting an organ removed and having an already depleted body blasted full of toxic, carcinogenic chemicals and radiation. It doesn't make a whole lot of sense, but those are the standard paradigms of our times.

There are obviously less dramatic ways to question and challenge the paradigms we have come to accept. We could talk about weight, for example. We follow a food pyramid that is supposed to guide our choices, try to

"We are stuck in an absurd cultural habit of thinking that medication will save us from lifestyle and social diseases."
– Dr. Mark Hyman

get the stories behind the photos http://bit.ly/UnDiet

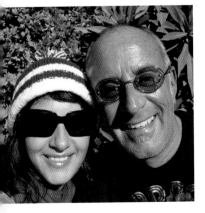

understand label claims, read magazine articles, and watch commercials on TV – but still 17 percent of American children aged two to nineteen are obese[3] and in 2008, 220,000 Americans elected to have gastric bypass surgery.[4] The numbers only grow as we continue to follow the current paradigms. Some may argue that if a child has two obese parents, the child is more likely to become obese. I question whether this is genetic or simply a diet and lifestyle inheritance. Regardless, just because we have the genetic switch, doesn't mean it needs to be turned on.

It seems easier to swallow a pill than make lifestyle changes. Cholesterol-lowering medications are among the top-selling pharmaceuticals in Canada and the United States[5] even though significant research has shown that these drugs do very little to decrease the risk of heart disease. What is missing from the medication equation is why cholesterol levels go up. If we ask this question, we question the protocol that is currently accepted. To do otherwise, to go outside the paradigm, would require change, and change is hard. In the immediate moment, it's often easier just to go with the flow than try and turn the current around, but just because that's the way the masses are flowing, doesn't make it the best way to go.

Approximately 88 percent of people over sixty are on some form of pharmaceutical medication. What's even more shocking is that 22 percent of children under the age of twelve are also on at least one prescribed medication.[6] Among children, the most common medications are for attention deficit disorder (ADD), with a higher concentration among boys than girls. Why are so many children having trouble sitting still and listening? Is it because they spend less time than they used to playing outside, burning off energy? Is it because a highly refined diet causes blood-sugar levels to rise and crash, causing symptoms of hyperactivity such as difficulty concentrating and mood instability? Are they inundated with the fast-moving pictures on television and computer games and not taught the skills of listening and patience? Or could it also be, in part, that kids are kids and part of wanting to express their innate kidness is to run around, make noise, play, and just express what they feel as they feel it?

Adult use of antidepressants almost tripled between 1988 and 2000.[7] Is it merely coincidence that in the mid- to late-nineties fat became the

villain in the diet? We all went fat-free, and with our egg-white omelets entered an epidemic of feeling funked out. Fat fuels the nervous system. Good
fats are what our brain is made of. We need fat to absorb fat-soluble vitamins. Vitamin D is a fat-soluble vitamin and Vitamin D deficiency is linked to
depression. Vitamin B3, or niacin, naturally found in all whole foods, and in
abundance in whole grains, helps alleviate depression, and B vitamins are
removed when our grains get processed from whole grains into white flour.
Our diet switched over to highly refined, nutrient-deficient processed ingredients – and our mood, libido, and zest for life went down the drain with
the egg yolk.

Prescriptions for nonsteroidal anti-inflammatory drugs, antidepressants,
blood glucose/sugar regulators and cholesterol-lowering statin drugs, in
particular, increased notably between 1996 and 2002.[8] These are prescribed
to help conditions that have their roots in diet and lifestyle choices. Additionally, standards of what constitutes high cholesterol, or defines depression, have
changed, with the threshold lowered so more people are being diagnosed with
more conditions and thereby being prescribed more medications.

That's a whole lot of pills, a whole lot of money, loads of side effects,
and we're not getting any healthier.

At what point do we ask if this paradigm is working? Does replacing a
microwave with a juicer still sound insane when people are popping expensive
pharmaceuticals daily without knowing what the long-term effects can be?

Sadly, this is not only limited to medications and disease states. Our
food system, as we know it, is becoming a worldwide threat to our health. So,
too, is the paradigm of mass food production. Transcontinental food recalls
are becoming commonplace.

*"We do not experience things as they really are! We experience
things only through a filter and that filter determines what
information will enter our awareness and what will be rejected.
If we change the filter (our belief system), then we automatically
experience the world in a completely different way."*
– David Wolfe

Have you ever had to look through your fridge and check SKUs or dates on your ground beef or processed luncheon meats? It is estimated that between 2007 and 2009 there were recalls of more than 45,000,000 pounds of beef.[9] This meat, from thousands of farms, gets shipped to a few major processors, then gets distributed across the globe and used in various processed forms. With the food-supply chain as it currently runs, there is no way to avoid major food-borne illness outbreaks. Your hamburger from your local fast-food drive-thru can contain parts from as many as one hundred different cows. One sickly little cow from one little farm can result in a massive worldwide problem.

What we all have to ask ourselves, as we move into the uncharted territory of the UnDiet is simple: Is what I am currently doing working for me? If your answer is anything other than a resounding *yes*, then it is time to make some changes.

You don't have to ditch the microwave and get the juicer, and you don't have to give up coffee all at once. We're doing this in baby steps. But if you are with me, riding beside me on the health train, then all aboard! We're pulling out of the station. It's time to move forward, break rules, and UnDiet to vibrant health.

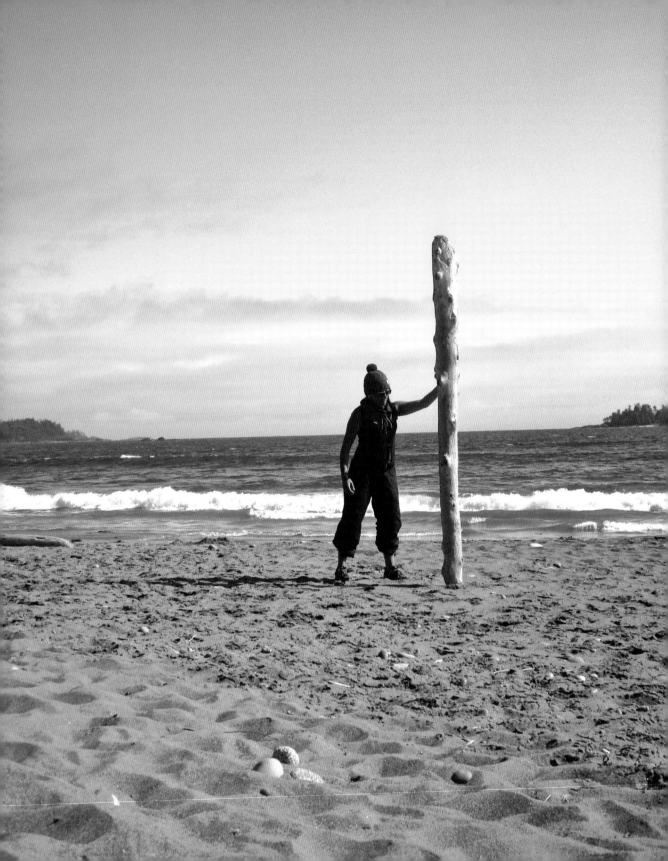

CHAPTER 2

The UnDiet Foundations

A DIET BUILT ON COUNTING CALORIES IS LIKE A MANSION BUILT ON SAND

A few years ago, I was visiting my grandma Fritzi in Winnipeg. She was eighty-seven at the time, and what she was eating for breakfast was not passing my evil nutrition eye unnoticed: a slice of rye bread and margarine with a cup of instant coffee. I wanted to make something special, so off to the health food store I went to pick up whole-food goodies to make up the very best granola.

She sat at the kitchen table watching me with a close eye as I put it all together. While the granola was lightly toasting, I chopped up some fresh fruit and scooped out plain organic yogurt. I served my grandma Fritzi a bowl of granola warm from the oven, complete with toasted oats, nuts, and seeds, a sprinkling of cinnamon and some raw honey with a dollop of yogurt and some fresh berries. My grandma looked at it with horror, asking, "What is that? A thousand calories?" I had to laugh and I asked her what a calorie was, a trick question for sure, as most people haven't a clue. My grandma's answer: "It's the fat you get from eating too many carbohydrates."

I would imagine that most people might guess something similar.

CALORIES DON'T COUNT

Calories are not the villain we make them out to be — always trying to cheat our way past them with foods that enable us to eat more in volume while consuming less in calories. If we eat calories above and beyond what we burn, no matter where they come from, all the extras get turned into junk in the trunk, or upper-arm wings, or inner-thigh squish. That's only half of it, though. It's the calorie-burning component that we fail to correctly take into account.

The basic flaw in a calorie-counting diet and most conventional diet programs, is that they rarely consider the nutritional value of the calorie. See, not all calories are created equal. Calories from sugar will do different things in the body than calories from fat. This means that calories from an apple, from an avocado, from a handful of gummy bears, or from a bowl of nachos will all function differently.

Just as not all calories are created equal, they also don't burn equally either. Calories are measured in labs, using this weird antiquated machine called the bomb calorimeter. Put on your white lab coat with me while I take you on a tour.

Inside the bomb calorimeter, electrical energy is used to ignite the fuel. In the case of calculating the calories in a food, the fuel is a food item. As the food burns, it will heat up the surrounding air, which runs through a tube into a basin of water. The water temperature increases and it is this increase that helps us calculate the calorie or energy count in the food. The measure of a calorie is the measure of how much energy is needed to raise 1 gram of water by 1 degree.

You can see then how a calorie count becomes a weird way to measure whether a food is good for us or not, right? Somehow, the measure of calories in a food is what most of us have come to base our food choices on. The tricky bit is that our stomachs are not bomb calorimeters. We do not burn up fuel the same way a machine does.

Therefore, when it comes to calories there are two main considerations to take into account.

* Our rate of burning calories will vary based on who we are, what we're doing, and the kinds of food we're eating.
* Not all calories are created equal.

Factors That Affect Calorie Burning

Instead of having a bomb calorimeter inside our bodies to which we can predictably feed fuel and measure its exact burning potential, we have something you may have heard of called metabolism. Unlike a big archaic machine with consistent water temperature measuring results, metabolism is variable. Some of the most common factors that can affect the efficiency of metabolism include:

* **Age:** Caloric needs vary at different ages, peaking around twenty-five and then declining by about 2 percent every ten years or so after that. This means we can almost eat what we want and get away with it until twenty-five, and then those pitchers of beer and late-night ice cream feasts catch up with us. As the body, ahem, matures, it is sadly more disposed to replacing muscle with fat without the right exercise and strength training. As we age, our metabolism, and as such, our calorie-burning potential, also slows down.

* **Sex:** This fun-filled activity speeds up metabolism, but what we're talking here is males versus females, not the bow-chica-bow variety. Men burn more calories than women. This is, for the most part, because men have less body fat and more muscle. The more muscle, the higher the metabolic rate, and the quicker the calories burn. As women tend not to have as much muscle mass as men, we need to kick up the cardio and include weight-bearing exercises to burn more calories. This changes during pregnancy and breastfeeding. Just when we need to get accustomed to one more weird

thing our body does, it decides to up and burn through calories like no-body's business. If you needed more reasons to breastfeed babies, let the increased metabolism be one more.

✽ **Heredity/Metabolic Type:** All living creatures burn through calories by the basic functions of living, such as keeping the heart beating and the lungs breathing. This basic resting metabolic rate is called the basal meta-bolic rate (BMR). The tricky bit with the equations to calculate your BMR is that there are different metabolic types. Some people have naturally faster metabolisms than others, and this also means that different people will thrive on different ratios of carbohydrates, fats, and proteins. Now this is more detail than we need to know at this point. What is important to under-stand right now is that all bodies are a one of a kind, therefore no two me-tabolisms are going to function in the same way.

✽ **The Condition of Your Body:** The shape and size of your body also affects how you burn calories. We are now clear that the more muscle we have the more calories we burn, and the more fat we have the fewer calories we burn. This is not to say that more muscle is better and more fat is worse – I believe in a little jiggle to go with the giggle – but it is important to find that place where you are healthy. Think of it this way: the body builder at the gym who has no neck because his shoulders and traps are so big could prob-ably burn through an ice cream a lot faster than that big guy who overflowed into your seat on your last cross-country flight. The paradox here is that the muscle man didn't get to be the muscle man by eating a lot of ice cream.

✽ **Activity Level:** The more active you are the more calories you burn. But you knew this already, right? The type of activity you choose, how long, how often, and what time of day will affect how you burn calories. Don't get hung up on the details here though. The key is really to find that time in the day when you will do it, and just do it!

✽ **Big, Bad Habits:** Who's been on the cigarette-and-coffee diet? For some reason people think this makes them skinny. Okay, sure; but also wrinkly, aged, stinky, and eventually cancerous. A ciggy and coffee will raise metabolism by 5 percent for about three hours. This equals a whopping thirteen calories. Enjoy those artificially sweetened, two-calorie breath mints to get rid of your bad-habit stench. You earned them!

✤ **Weather:** Don't we love to blame the weather? Now we get to blame our lazy metabolism on it, or perhaps thank it. We can burn more calories when we're shivering timbers. The contraction and relaxation of muscles is the body's way of producing heat in order to maintain a steady body temperature. It's not just the cold, though; during hot summer nights, we burn through more calories by sweating. When the temperature is moderate, neither extremely hot or cold, and without activity, the metabolism rests at your basal metabolic rate.

✤ **The Powers of the Mind:** Sorry kiddies, we can't think our way to a fast metabolism. We can, however, worry our way to one. Stress and anxiety can cause a rapid increase in energy expenditure. When we go into a fight-or-flight mode, different chemicals circulate in the blood vessels and send an SOS to the cells that this is a dire state of affairs and it's time to break down energy stores in order to provide a greater supply of energy if needed. Don't go thinking in some twisted way that worry and stress are serving you. Any increase in metabolism from stress is likely balanced by an increase in other stress hormones that add to the old muffin top around the waistline – and an increased consumption of chocolate bars.

Not All Calories Are Created Equal

Given that we've relinquished all responsibility for the way our bodies look on the inside and outside to our team of doctors, aestheticians, trainers, nutritionists, hair stylists, and Botox injectors, wouldn't it also be great to have someone else tell us what we should be eating? That's what those little nutrition labels on the sides of boxes and the health claims splashed across them attempt to do for us. Or, rather, what we let them do. We like to think that if we do the correct math, add up our approximate 2,000 calories per day, or maybe even calculate that to lose two pounds per week we need to cut back on *X* calories per day, or increase our activity level by *Y* amount, then we'll be slick and sleek and bikini-ready by that holiday three months from now. Oh my dear love, sweet lovers, what a grand place that would be – grand if you like feeling deprived, hungry, and bored by every meal.

Just as I talked about how there are various factors that can affect how we burn our calories, we also have to know very clearly that not all calories are created equal and if health was simply a matter of consuming the magic number's worth, there'd be no need for an UnDiet, or gastric-bypass surgeries, or *Diabetic Living* magazine.

Let's take, for example, a 200-calorie snack. If you wanted to have a 200-calorie snack, you could choose between any of the following:

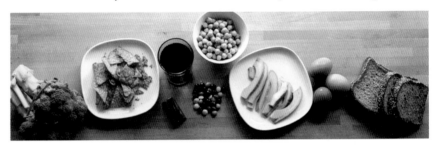

When we pull out our calculators at mealtime, we often forget that different calories in different forms will do different things inside our body and affect our metabolism in different ways.

Ever hear the term "empty calories"? An empty-calorie snack would be that handful of chips or the candies. You get caloric content in the form of hydrogenated oils in the case of the chips and in the form of refined sugar with the candies, but there is zero real nutritional value. It's even worse than zero, as these highly refined, highly processed foods will actually deplete your body of vital nutrients. The result is an excess of calories and a deficiency in nutrition, resulting in more cravings.

Empty-calorie foods lack the vital nutrients that the body needs to run optimally. High-sugar foods slow the metabolism right down to a sluggish, fat-storing mode. Even though those point-system diets may value an apple and a cookie as the same, as they have an equal quantity of calories, the quality is very different: one is packed with nutrients and the other completely void. Think of the apple as the high-octane fuel in the tank and the cookies as sand. The apple will help run that engine in our bodies along that windy scenic landscape, and the cookie will cause us to crash and burn out. When a package says the food contained within has zero calories from fat, do you know what that means? Not a whole lot. It means that the calories in that packaged food come from other sources, usually carbohydrates and usually in the form of sugar. Calorie intake, above and beyond what we burn, no matter if the source is protein, carbohydrates or fat, will all turn to fat on the body if not burned.

A high intake of calories from sugar can, in some cases, be more harmful to health than calories from fat. Calories from refined sugar require very little digestion time. This means that they will rush the blood stream, the pancreas will secrete bucketloads of insulin to try and get that sugar into the cells, and what can't be processed fast enough will be converted to fat. Calories from good fats – the unprocessed, cold-pressed variety – will absorb more slowly, at a rate that allows our cells to burn them more efficiently, and so less is converted to fat.

Carbohydrates, **protein**, and fat
ALL CONTAIN CALORIES,
in the following measures:

Protein: 4 calories/gram

Carbohydrates: 4 calories/gram

Fat: 9 calories/gram

Alcohol: 7 calories/gram

There is a basic ratio we need to abide by to maintain a healthy weight relating to calories in versus calories out, but the vital component we are forgetting is consideration for the building blocks that make up those calories. What is the actual goodness contained naturally in the foods we're choosing?

Toss the calculator. Remove that math equation from the plate. The only thing we'll be counting in the UnDiet is the thousands of ways we are looking and feeling better.

THE GOOD, THE BAD AND THE POISON: MACRO VERSUS MICRO NUTRIENTS

It is a blessed thing that, if you are reading this, you might also have a fridge full of food (or it would be if you'd left work early enough to get to the store), and enjoy an occasional meal out with friends.

Do you know, though, how many people are going hungry? Like, really starving? I am not referring to horrible situations in far-off lands or here at home with kids not getting breakfasts and families having to budget food stamps, though that too is a problem and a very similar one. What I am referring to is the fact that most of us are starving for nutrition.

The problem is not necessarily relegated to socioeconomics, meaning it's not completely defined by what people can *afford* to eat, but more so by what people *choose* to eat. And for the most part, our choices have led us to a developed world where people are dramatically overfed and severely undernourished.

As a society, we are not suffering from deficiencies in carbohydrates, protein, and fat. We are getting more than enough, hence the rising rates of obesity, type 2 diabetes (formerly referred to as "adult onset" until children started developing this condition), heart disease, high cholesterol, and a whole cocktail of conditions that have become commonplace. Metabolic syndrome, a prime example, is a condition where the organs and systems of the body begin to shut down. This condition was identified only twenty years ago and referred to simply as "Syndrome X." The thing about metabolic syndrome is that it is not a disease unto itself but a collection of symptoms or conditions that include: high blood pressure, imbalanced blood sugar, unhealthy cholesterol levels, and abdominal fat. Currently, over 40 percent of Americans between sixty and sixty-nine years of age[1] and 39 percent of Canadians between seventy and seventy-nine years of age[2] suffer from metabolic syndrome — a condition completely preventable by right living. For the most part, these conditions are a collection of symptoms attributed to an excessive intake of carbs, fats, and proteins combined with severe nutrient deficiency.

Carbohydrates, protein, and fat are what we call *macronutrients*. They are the big guys that make up the majority of the food we eat; the nutrients that get all the attention. What we often fail to pay attention to is the *micronutrient* value of our food. This is where nutrient deficiency comes in. Micronutrients are what the body needs to function optimally and healthfully. These include the vitamins, minerals, essential fats, phytonutrients (plant-derived nutrients that are essential to sustaining life), antioxidants, enzymes, fiber, water, and other synergistic properties that naturally occur in whole unprocessed foods. They are the main keys that our body uses to fuel our cells, and the tissues, organs, and organ systems made up of those cells that are required to run our body. This is where the concept of overfed and undernourished comes in to play. We are eating more than our share in calories from the macronutrients (fats, carbs, and proteins), and continue to starve for nutrition from the micronutrients – the actual elements needed to optimally operate the systems that fuel our body. Those key micronutrients are where we are lacking – and what 70 percent of the population seemingly prefer to take in the form of daily supplements.[3]

This is where the idea of macronutrients versus micronutrients comes in. The macronutrients are the things we like to look out for on the back of our breakfast cereal box. These are the components of our diet that have turned our mealtimes into math equations. Focusing on these basic factors has caused much of the population to become very fat, very sick, and dramatically depleted in vital, health sustaining micronutrients. In a 2007–2009 study, Statistics Canada found that 37 percent of the population is classified as overweight, with an additional 24 percent classified as obese.[4] As of 2010, 34 percent of Americans were categorized as obese.[5]

Calories alone are not an indication of whether something is healthy. They may be a fun thing for us to add up, but in the grand scheme of things, when it comes to the actual health value of our food, calories don't count. For example, fat is more calorically dense, gram for gram, than the other macronutrients, but if from a good source, they are also nutritionally dense, high in micronutrients, and we therefore need less to feel satiated.

Just as not all calories are created equal, neither are the macronutrients. We can eat foods that are high in fat, that have no nutritional power punch, like a doughnut, or we can eat foods high in fat, like an avocado, that can function as a perfect multivitamin. One of these is going to drain the tank and the other will fuel the vehicle of our body and our life. I'll let you consider that one.

What we want to look for then, as we break into this UnDieted great, food-loving way of living, is choosing foods that are the most concentrated in terms of the micronutrients for every bite of the macronutrient. These are going to be things such as green leafy vegetables; non-starchy vegetables; beans, lentils, and legumes; fresh fruit; whole grains, nuts, and seeds; sea vegetables; and lean meats, fish, and eggs. And of course, if you want to rock this out totally veg style, go for it my plant-loving sistas and brothas.

Fat is Fat: All fat has the same caloric content whether it is butter, extra virgin olive oil, or processed margarine. Since fat is essential for brain and nervous system health, you're better off eating the very best quality you can get. Hint: it's not going to be a processed butter-like product.

Nutrient Density Chart

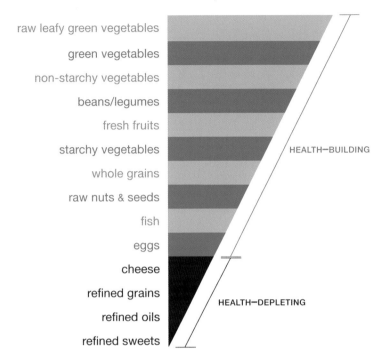

raw leafy green vegetables
green vegetables
non-starchy vegetables
beans/legumes
fresh fruits
starchy vegetables
whole grains
raw nuts & seeds
fish
eggs
cheese
refined grains
refined oils
refined sweets

HEALTH—BUILDING

HEALTH—DEPLETING

When we get out of the habit of counting weird stuff like calories from fat, grams of carbs, and the daily ratio of protein intake, and just start choosing most of our food from the unprocessed, nutrient-dense realm, all the math starts to take care of itself. We can put the abacus away and get back to cooking, eating, loving, laughing, and totally and completely thriving on the foods we eat.

Imagine how life would be if you woke up every morning feeling fantabulous. You hop out of bed with a skip in your step, craving your morning green juice, knowing an award-winning poop was to follow, with time to exercise and meditate before your work day begins. Your energy, mood, concentration, calmness, and clarity rocks with you all day long. And then, the most amazing thing would happen at the end of the day – you would enjoy a great meal, max and relax, and when it came time to go to sleep, you get into bed, close your eyes, and not wake up until the morning. How different would your life be?

Your body feels great to be in, as do your jeans, but that's not the focus here. When we eat what we need, as opposed to what our emotions and imbalances cause us to crave and binge on, we have the energy for the right amount of exercise and our bodies will naturally slim on down or curve on out to where they are happiest and feel the most balanced.

This is how the UnDiet revolution leads us to vibrant health.

Building Health or Building Disease?

This quickly becomes the almighty question. We obviously don't ever want to think that we have had a personal hand in the development of our chronic headaches, monthly pre-period weep-athons, inability to keep on or lose weight, or the low libido that keeps us from getting it on with our lover. Sorry, but we have to. We have to think about it and we have to take responsibility.

Everything we've done up until this very point in time has contributed to our current state of health. This isn't just about the foods we eat, but also the places we work, the amount we sleep, how often we exercise, how we engage and respond to others in our life, how much we love sharing our life with that special someone, how deeply we breathe, how much time we spend on the computer or in the car, right down to the thoughts we think.

Let's collectively agree, right now, even if your boss is a monkeyball and your upstairs neighbors seem to walk around with bricks on their feet, that you are going to own it all. The good with the bad. Own it.

We're not going to *ohm* on that, or call a girlfriend for a woman-powered cry-a-thon. Let's just move forward, accepting that our shit is our own and making sure that the big old wheel of life keeps turning. That means we're going to keep rolling with it, but moving forward we'll roll with it while wearing a touch of a smile on our face and a sense of empowerment in our heart. Allow me to explain.

"You have everything you need to build something far bigger than yourself."
– Seth Godin

Disease, for the most part, is built in the body. We don't catch a cold, not really. We have built the conditions, like lack of sleep, poor stress management, sugar or alcohol intake, or low nutrient intake, that create the ideal environment for that germ to grab hold inside and turn our noses into faucets. We also don't catch a big booty, type 2 diabetes, or heart disease. These things are not contagious, but are slow-growing, slow-building conditions. It can be argued that there are communicable diseases that can be contracted, and that some people are more prone to certain things than others, but when it all comes down to it, as Louis Pasteur proclaimed on his deathbed, "The pathogen is nothing; the terrain is everything."

It is possible, if we live strong and healthy lives, that we can be immune to all kinds of conditions believed to be both contagious, such as the flu, and degenerative, such as tooth decay, cataracts, arthritis, and heart disease, to name a few. If we can agree that we have to own our health, and our current state is a result of the choices we've made in our sweet life so far, then we also have to accept that some of those choices have influenced the healthy bits of us, and some worked toward those areas that might need a little more care.

In short, everything we eat, breathe, think, or do will either build our health or build our disease. There isn't a lot of gray area in this.

It can be said that foods that are good for our spirit are good for our health. This is where chocolate cake in the spirit of celebration might come in. Chocolate cake shared with friends in celebration of you being amazing is quite different than bingeing on a frozen processed chocolate cake, eaten out of the freezer at midnight while tears stream down your face, only to be chased by feelings of remorse and guilt. Negative emotion will do far more harm to our health than a slice of cake ever could. But of course you also must remember that all "in the spirit of celebration" indulgences should ideally be partaken in with the utmost selectivity. Nourishing your spirit with chocolate cake every night of the week is called building disease or bad habits. It's also the ultimate act of disrespect to your fair and beautiful self.

Suddenly, all the complicated measures we've used in our lives to decide what we should or should not do gets narrowed down to a simple question: will this work toward my goals or against them? Easy as that. The next time you're jonesing for that processed faux-milk, candy-topped, ice-cream treat from the local drive-thru, ask yourself that question. When ordering from the menu at your fave resto-lounge when you're dining late into the night, you can ask that question.

I guarantee you will always, *always* know the right answer. Listening to that voice inside your head, which may start to sound a bit like mine, will be the tougher part. I figure though, if you follow it 85 percent of the time, maybe 70 percent, or even just 60 percent, you're still doing better than not doing anything at all. Every little bit is going to help. Bringing awareness, a

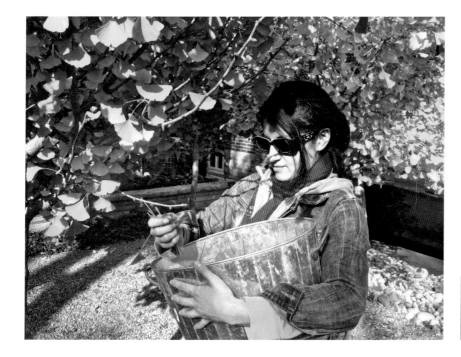

get the stories
behind the photos
http://bit.ly/UnDiet

sense of mindfulness or consciousness, to your choices as they relate to what you eat will extend to other bits of your life, including your work and love life. You become more aware of everything and how it makes you feel. The result of this awareness is that the next time we're faced with that same decision – whether it be what to order off that menu or whether that hot tamale deserves a second date – our decisions become based on what will build us up both in the short term, as well as for the long haul. When you start feeling absolutely and totally amazing, you are less tempted to choose things on the disease-building side of life.

And now, my love, I do believe that together we are ready to embark on the life-changing, amped-up, life-loving, food-eating adventure that will break the rules, bring love into the kitchen, and bring you vibrant health. It is time to UnDiet.

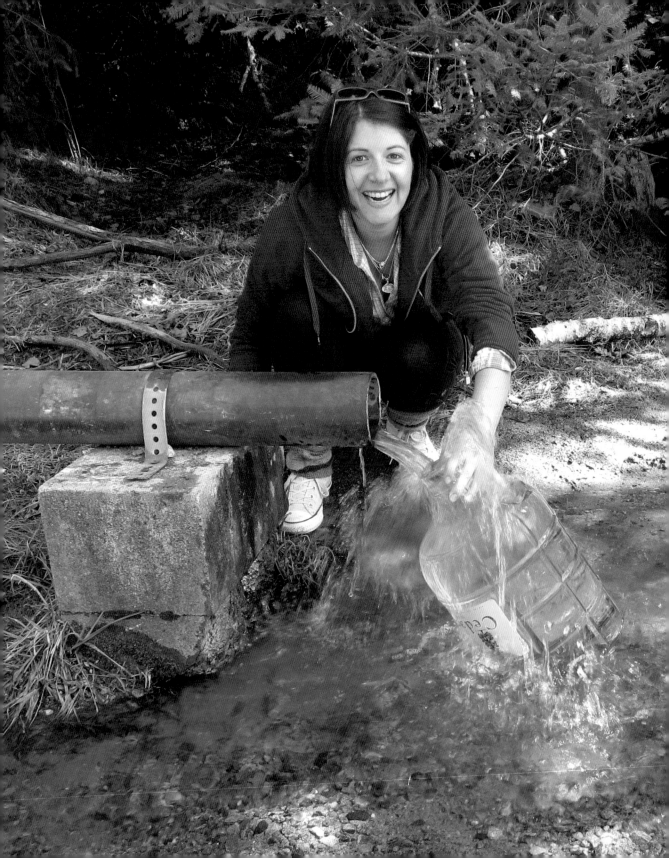

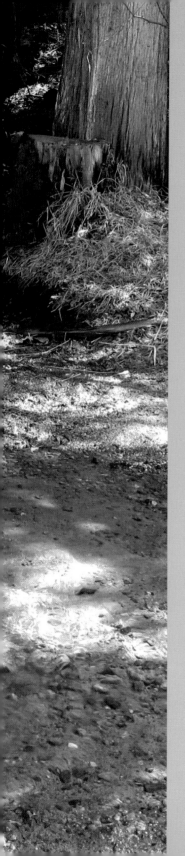

CHAPTER 3

Start Sipping

We're going to start off easy like Sunday morning. It's time to quench that long-forgotten thing we call thirst. We often fail to notice how thirsty we are until our hands are like pieces of sandpaper, our lips are chapped, our joints are creaky, and we're wondering how we used up that tube of lube beside the bed so quickly. Or maybe it's when we feel thirsty enough to gulp down a gallon in a single long sip. Same thing. Proper hydration is going to affect every single part of us that requires moisture in order to function, from brain to belly to libido.

WHY HYDRATE?

The body depends on just the right amount of hydration for survival. It doesn't get much more basic than that. Every cell, tissue, and organ of the body needs water to function and the more fresh and clean water we get down, the more efficiently every process in the body is going to operate. Water makes up 75 percent of all muscle and 23 percent of fatty tissue. That's pretty much most of the body. The body uses water to maintain its temperature, to digest food, to cleanse cells, and to eliminate waste. We lose water in all kinds of ways, such as breathing, sweating, exercising, and sexing. Are you a chatterbox or does your job requires you to talk a lot? Then you need more water too.

Thirst versus Hunger

Top water-dense foods

Cucumber ✔
Watermelon ✔
Celery ✔
Apples ✔
Romaine ✔
Citrus fruits ✔

Most of us are not getting enough of the sweet nectar from the springs of our planet. We're simply not drinking enough, and not eating enough foods high in water content.

The brain plays a tricky little game on us with this whole thirst versus hunger thing. It gets confused and it's not to our advantage. It is very rare that we'll get the message, *My oh my, I am hungry, let me just drink a glass or gallon of water and see how I feel after*. But it is very possible that we get a thirst signal, and somehow it gets confused in translation and we think, *My oh my, I am hungry, let me go eat that bag of potato chips and see how I feel after.*

Top dehydrating foods

Alcohol ✘
Coffee ✘
Soda pop ✘
Deep-fried anything ✘
Refined bread ✘
Crackers ✘
Chips ✘

We usually won't notice that we're thirsty until we feel a dry mouth or throat. At this point, dehydration has already set in. The problem is that when we get dehydrated, our energy level will drop. The brain sends out the signals for energy and most of us answer this call not by checking our thirst, but by grabbing the nearest bit of grub that can give us quick energy. The result is that we are treating the *symptoms* of dehydration – the energy drop – rather than the *cause* – the need for good, clean, plain water.

Sipping on Calories

I know I already went through this whole thing with you about how calories don't count, but we're about breaking rules here and there is one place where calories absolutely do count – when it comes to our drinks. Calories through a straw are still calories in and in the form of soda, fruit juice, and booze those calories are bad to the mineral-stripped bone.

Most of the added sugar in our lives comes through the straw. On average we consume 22 teaspoons of added sugar a day – that's about 350 calories and at least half of that is in drinkable form from fruit juices that line super-market aisles, those sickly sweet sodas, and the barfiest of all inventions, strawberry flavored milk.[1] Those 350 extra calories per day work out to 2,450 extra calories per week. That's like a whole extra day of eating!

Even a freshly pressed apple, grape, orange, and mango glass-of-heaven juice isn't the best choice. All fruit, when consumed as fruit, is amazingly delicious and great for us, but when we get to juicing, we're separating out the juicey bits from the fibery bits, leaving the sugar content free and clear to surge our blood stream. Without the fiber, all that sugar, despite being naturally occurring, is going to spike the blood sugar. We then move into the territory of sugar spikes, insulin spikes, slowing metabolism, expanded waistlines, and the imbalanced hormones that follow.

Does Coffee and a Martini Count As Water?

When I was in university, I had a boyfriend who spent his days drinking coffee and his nights drinking pitchers of beer. Fairly standard practice for university gents. Sadly, most people carry these horrific habits into their adult lives and wind up with all sorts of grossness going on in their bodies – starting with the brightest, most foul-smelling pee. This, my sweet sipper, is a sure sign that you're dehydrated.

Caffeinated drinks, which include coffee, black tea, green tea, energy drinks, and sodas, have an extremely dehydrating effect on the body. So does alcohol. The technical term here is diuretic. This is an action of a food, herb, or in this case, a drink that stimulates your kidneys to increase the excretion of sodium in the urine. When the kidneys excrete sodium, they excrete water from the blood along with it – flushing out vital nutrients. With alcohol, the body is just trying to get this out as fast as possible. Hence, more water out of the blood through the kidneys and less water in the body.

Thirsty? For every caffeinated or alcoholic beverage consumed, you must rehydrate with at least two glasses of plain water.

Does this mean you have to give up all those coffees, teas, and drink nights with the ladies? Not necessarily. We're UnDieting here and deprivation never got anyone to abundance. What it does mean is that you have to be aware,

KEEP THE ICE OUT OF THE GLASS When we drink icy cold water, it causes the blood vessels in our stomach to contract, thus becoming less absorbent. This will slow the hydration process. Additionally, icy cold water requires enzyme activity in the body to help heat it up until it is around body temperature. This slows down the hydration process and also uses up a whole lot of enzyme action that is likely better used to help us digest our food. And the last big boo on ice cold water – when consumed while eating a meal, it will completely slow the digestive process, causing poor breakdown of food, contributing to indigestion and poor nutrient absorption.

conscious, and mindful about your intake. A half-dozen coffees a day is far too many, as is drinking a whole pitcher of beer or a triple threat of martinis.

I can hear you yelling at me right now. Stop it. It's for your own good. And I know what you're thinking, too – that if you normally have three cups of coffee before noon, that means drinking six glasses of water which totals nine beverages. You're afraid you'll be running back and forth to the bathroom a thousand times. And you're right. You will be. So don't drink so much coffee, or be grateful for the extra exercise. The choice is yours.

What we often don't think about is how proper hydration can actually kick our energy and concentration ability into high gear. Sip up, think better, move faster. Booyah!

JUST DRINK THE WATER

Through your refined skills of deduction, you have likely come to the conclusion that as we UnDiet to the life of our dreams, we'll be drinking loads of water and not much else. You would be correct, my fair, water-loving mermaid. If we revisit the concept of foods that work toward our goals and those that work against us, where would canned iced teas, ginger ale, and a frozen-mocha-coffee treat fall?

I will remind you that this doesn't mean you can't meet up with your best lady-love girlfriends for a half-caff-mocha-latte-skinna-marinky-dinky-do when the weather is warm, or fill your home with the aromas of a fresh brewed cup of coffee or tea on a lazy Sunday morning, but these are not your everyday lovers; they're more like conjugal visitors. You can see them only once in a while and you'd best make the most of your time together. I can almost guarantee that in time, you'll be ready to part ways with your past exploits as you discover new delights.

Ten Best Reasons to Drink Loads of Water

Crank That Energy Crunk. Don't even start to tell me how tired you feel every day. Everyone is always tired! When was the last time you were on an airplane? People are zonked out and head-mamboing within twenty-seven seconds of takeoff. Water is an important part of the energy equation. It only takes the itty-bittiest bit of dehydration to slow down the action of the enzymes in our body that keeps our cellular energy-making activity high and mighty. Without the enzyme activity, fatigue begins to set in. Forget about having the motivation to go for a walk or exercise in any other way. In short, keeping that thirst quenched will help keep your energy up.

1

Get Metabolizing, Absorbing, and Pooping. Proper hydration is vital to each and every stage of the digestive process. Interesting factoid: our bodies produce an average of 1.75 gallons of digestive juices daily. Do you know what is needed to make up those 1.75 gallons? It's not diet soda and lattes, that's for sure. If we don't drink enough water, we are unable to produce the juices we need to break the goods down. Without breakdown or metabolizing the food we eat, we are less able to absorb the nutrients in our food. Hello indigestion, pull up a curve of the small intestine and stay for a while.

2

Now, that is water's effect in the upper or first part of digestion. Down below, in the large colon, we need enough water to bulk up the fiber we consume. It creates a little sponge scenario. We need that bulk, combined with proper hydration, to get the waste out effectively and efficiently. Under times of dehydration, we can't get it out, and the body starts to reabsorb the moisture, or what I call "poo juice," that is in the stool. That's where constipation starts to kick in. We feel like we have to go and all we get for our efforts are little rabbit-pellet poops. As you may well know, being bunged up makes you feel icky and knowing that this is caused by dehydration and the reabsorption of poo juice should be enough motivation for you to go and have some water right now.

3 Immune-Boosting Power Party. Water is vital for helping flush waste matter from the body. Part of this waste originates in the diet, and much of what is eliminated is from our previous day's food intake. That's not the only source, though. There is also waste matter in the form of toxins that enter our body from the products we use on our skin, the air we breathe, and the by-products of regular metabolism. Water is vital for flushing the cells of this waste build-up. If we're not hydrated, we're not flushing – our cells or the loo!

Back to the pooping component for a moment: When we aren't flushing our cells of toxins, and then not properly eliminating those toxins from our body, we end up carrying that waste around with us all day. It slows down our overall metabolic functioning and can cause chronic aches and pains, headaches, menstrual problems, allergies, and an all-around heavy feeling. When elimination is not regular, from the cells themselves or from the body as a whole, we become more inflamed and toxic, weakening the immune system and making us more susceptible to infection and illness, not to mention creating a prime environment for slow-building diseases such as cancer.

4 Keep the Blood Flowing Free. It is true that our blood is made of protein and that we need those good fats from fish, nuts, and seeds, and also antioxidants like vitamin E to keep the blood flowing, but we also need good old water, too. When in a state of chronic dehydration, our blood becomes thicker and stickier. The body always does its best to repair the havoc we wreak on it, and in this case, the body attempts to keep things moving by working harder to push that blood through the veins. The result is that blood pressure goes up. Drinking water and staying hydrated is a great first line of defense against high blood pressure and so much better than pills, many of which list dehydration and its symptoms as side effects.

5 Cholesterol Showdown. Cholesterol is a fatty substance found in the blood, produced in every cell of the body and is the parent hormone for all the other hormones we produce – a bit like the master puppeteer. Despite our wide-spread belief that cholesterol is an evil villain, it serves many essential functions and at healthy levels is vital for health. Cholesterol levels tend to rise in response to high toxic load, emotional or physical trauma, high free-radical circulation, and inflammation. As it relates to hydration, cholesterol helps form part of the membrane around each and every cell of our bodies. It keeps our cells, including those in our skin, waterproof. Without it, we'd be spilling out. For the most part, cholesterol is not a dietary issue but a symptom or response in the body to other things that are going on. When we are dehydrated, water content or moisture is naturally drawn out of the cells by the process of osmosis (wanting balance on both sides of the gate). In an attempt to protect the coveted holy grail of the cell (the DNA), the cells will produce more cholesterol to strengthen the cell membrane and protect the cell from further dehydration. The result, however, is often not just a thickening of the cell membranes but this cholesterol will also pour into the blood stream, thus contributing to elevated cholesterol levels. Now aren't you glad we cleared the air around this one?

Management of the Junk in Your Trunk. Though we know for sure that skinny doesn't automatically equal healthy, we also know that carrying too much weight is not a good thing. Since you're now versed in how our brains can confuse thirst and hunger, I will just summarize here. When we're dehydrated, we feel tired, and this feeling is often confused with a need for fuel. Eating food can essentially soothe feelings of thirst and fatigue caused by dehydration. The function of this can lead to false sensations of hunger that can cause the mindless munchies, resulting in overeating. The junk in the trunk isn't always fat, either. Cellulite is not a curse bestowed on women by some mean cottage cheese–hating master of thighs. It is a sign of built up toxins in fat cells. Toxins love to snuggle away in our fat cells and our bums are ripe with snuggling material. Poor hydration thereby can increase the amount of toxins we store in our cells, thus contributing to cottage-cheese thighs (cellulite). Dehydration can also increase circulating inflammatory compounds. All of this adds digits on to our scale reading, too.

Such a Pretty Face. It's true that a face can be stretched, tucked, lifted and injected, but the skin itself rarely lies. Without proper hydration, it starts to sag. It loses elasticity and gets all dry and flaked out. Grossness factor. Ever heard the saying, "The solution for pollution is dilution"? To get the toxins out, we need to sweat. In order to sweat properly, we need enough hydration to act as the vehicle to sweat stuff out. Dehydration doesn't allow toxins to be adequately diluted for easy removal. We actually need to sweat about twenty-four ounces a day to properly flush out and eliminate the toxins we store as well as those that are created as natural byproducts of the body's metabolic processes. Without adequate hydration, the crap will store up in our cells until, eventually, it starts busting out of our face and armpits in the form of pimply complexions and stinky body odor.

8

Dropping Acid. The tissues of the body have a pH level, which is a measure of acidity and alkalinity. Ideally, the score of a resting body hangs out in the slightly alkaline range of 7.4 on the pH scale. The more acidic your body is, the more prone you are to all kinds of pathogens, fungi, bacteria, and inflammation. Consuming a less than stellar amount of water slows down the production and activity of enzymes, which are needed to keep the processes of the body in motion. The slower the motion, the more acidic the body environment becomes. Other things that create a more acid environment, by the way, includes poor digestion, constipation, and drinking sweet drinks. It's an evil mix.

9

Internal Lubing. Joints, cartilage, and ligaments that are dried out like a rice cake are far more brittle and therefore prone to injury. To add insult to injury, literally, any kind of injury that results in inflammation will create circulating inflammatory compounds that can aggravate other conditions. Then there's the old dry vagina problem that plagues women both young and old. The base of female lubricant is water. Drink it up so you can have a good time. The lube that keeps all of our joints, ligaments, and coochies slip sliding with ease into old age has to come from somewhere. Water is a perfect thing to help that along.

10

Age Is Just a Number. . . . Unless of course your face looks like a used leather handbag. A normal aging process happens due to the gradual loss in cell volume – think of a grape drying out into a raisin. The cells just start to deflate. This deflation into old wrinkle-bottom is accelerated with a life of caffeine, booze, and sugar – all things that dehydrate us. Drinking water is the surest way to slow down the aging process and keep our skin looking plump and youthful. How we look on the outside will give us a good idea of the state of our cells on the inside. Used leather handbag on the outside, used leather handbag on the inside. And one other thing: Botox and plastic surgery may seem like an easy option to look younger, but 1) most often people wind up looking totally weird and 2) isn't drinking water just a wee bit easier (and cheaper)?

EIGHT MOST DELIGHTFUL WAYS TO MAKE DRINKING WATER FABULOUS

Now that you're sold on drinking water to your heart and thirst's content to keep the toxic waste flushing out, your blood swimming along, your energy up, and your face as smooth as a baby's tush, let's make it fun. Drinking water doesn't have to be the drabbity-drab boringness we often think. Here are the best ways to jazz up this nectar from Mamma Earth:

❋ **Sliced Cucumber:** Just like being at the spa. Let the cukes soak in your water and while sipping, turn on some ocean sounds, then fish out the cuke slices and throw them over your eyes. Yes, just like being at the spa.

❋ **Essential Oils:** Making sure you're rocking the food-grade goodies, essential oils will liven up your water and enhance your health too. Lavender will be calming; tangerine, sweet and tangy; and mint to energize and also calm digestive upset. One drop is plenty.

❋ **Aloe Leaf:** Fresh aloe leaf (yes like the one you have sitting in your sunny window) has a hydrophilic quality, meaning it attracts water. Chop one tablespoon up and let it sit in a glass of water. Drink it all up and feel the cleansing hydration take hold. Be adventurous and eat up the aloe pulp after, but you may want to stay close to a loo – it can be cleansing.

❋ **Ginger Root:** A thumb-size slice of fresh ginger root will lightly infuse your water, fight off any nausea or nerves, and promote digestion.

The Solution is Dilution: If you're still craving that glass of fruit juice or even soda, dilute it with water (even bubbly). Start by diluting by 25 percent, then 50 percent, and then only add a splash of juice to what you're drinking. You'll soon be shocked by how sweet that drink is in its full strength.

❋ **Watermelon:** Sweeten the loving naturally with a little watermelon, chilled or frozen — and a packet of watermelon-flavored artificial ingredients is not the same thing.

❋ **Frozen Grapes:** You're not filling your glass with these frozen gems and then adding a bit of water; you're adding two or three frozen grapes. A little treat at the end of the glass.

❋ **Sliced Lemon:** An old favorite. Adds a little flavor, a vitamin C boost, and makes it look fancy-pants.

❋ **Accessorize:** A pretty glass and delightful glass straw, along with a sweet pitcher sitting on your desk, will make sipping water feel like a decorative indulgence all day long. Make it look glam and sip more in the process.

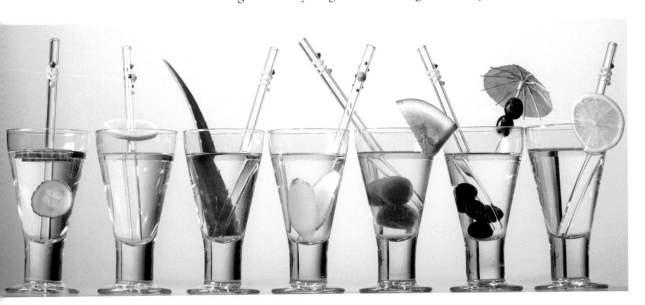

WHAT ELSE ARE WE DRINKING?

I get it. Once in a while you want a break from always being on the water. I'm with you on this. There are many options you can turn to in those moments of wanting some *oomph*.

❀ **Green Juice:** Green juices, meaning juices made from predominantly green vegetables, are not the same as fruit juices. For the most part, they are going to have way less sugar. One of the reasons we want to keep fruit juices at bay is because of the high concentration of sugar that will flood your body without the whole fruit form fiber intact (as it does in a whole fruit) to slow it down. This same function, however, is what makes low-sugar green juices so amazing. What you get with a green juice is a massive concentration of nutrients – vitamins, minerals, phytonutrients, and enzymes with low amounts of sugars, as green veggies don't have much to begin with. We are then able to quench our thirst, keep our blood sugar stable, and flood our body with the greatest detoxification elixir there ever was, not to mention an abundance of enzymes to keep the metabolic motion in action.

Mix and Match Your Green Blend

FRUIT/VEGETABLE	BENEFIT[2,3]
Apple	Works to prevent Alzheimer's and Parkinson's disease.
Beet	Assists detoxification and fights inflammation.
Bok Choy	Great for skin and cardiovascular health.
Broccoli	Supports the body through the detox process, reduces inflammation.
Cabbage	Heals stomach lining and peptic ulcers, regulates stomach bacteria.
Carrot	Helps treat acne and other skin problems.
Celery	Lowers blood pressure.
Cilantro	Removes heavy metals, is anti-inflammatory, and lowers blood sugar.
Collard Greens	Potent anti-aging effects.
Cranberry	Prevents urinary tract infections.
Cucumber	Fights kidney, bladder, liver, and pancreatic diseases.
Dandelion Greens	Improves liver function and circulation.
Ginger	Good for digestion, nausea, and reducing inflammation
Kale	Amps up body's detoxification system to clear out toxic substances.
Lemon	Tones the liver, cleanses the cells.
Parsley	Boosts immune system, prevents against infections and colds.
Romaine Lettuce	Helps prevent neural-tube birth defects in the beginning stages of pregnancy.
Spinach	Helps control colon, lung, and breast cancers.

❋ **Herbal Teas:** Cutting our fluorescent-colored drinks doesn't mean you have to go all grandma on me and start sipping chamomile 24/7. There is much in between as far as herbal teas go, and with fancy-shmancy tea bars popping up all over the place, discovering new blends to fall in love with has never been more fun or trendy. Herbal tea, more accurately called a tisane, is a steeping of various herbs in hot water, as opposed to the brewing of tea leaves, which is what a tea is, if you want to get official. Different herbs will have different effects on your mind, mood, and energy. A super fun thing to do is to work out what herbs have benefits that may help your woes, mixed with some you like just because they're delicious, and create your own, from-scratch, herbal tea blends. I know you'll kind of fancy being a professional tea blender because it's so fun. Don't go thinking you need to head over to your local apothecary for this either, though you might want to; many of the best herbs for brewing your own tea are already sitting on your spice rack (or should be!).

Create an Herbal Tea Blend All Your Own

HERB	HEALTH EFFECT[4]
Anise	Aids in digestion, acts as a decongestant, and has calming effects.
Cardamom	Helps in conditions of indigestion as well as reducing nausea and vomiting, soothes menstrual pain, reduces excess phlegm in coughs and colds.
Catnip	Mild sedative effect that helps with insomnia, anxiety, general nervousness; eases digestive complaints; antifungal.
Chamomile	Strengthens the immune system, therefore helps fight infections, eases muscles spasms and inflammation, soothes nerves, and promotes relaxation.
Cinnamon	Useful for balancing blood sugar, enhances circulation, aphrodisiac, eases digestive discomfort.
Fennel	Reduces digestive spasms and farts, eases symptoms of coughs and colds.
Fenugreek	Balances blood sugar levels, improves digestion, improves kidney function.
Ginger	Calms digestive discomfort (especially nausea), decreases inflammation (especially arthritis), reduces symptoms of allergies and colds.

Gingko Biloba	Enhances circulation, improves memory and alertness, reduces fatigue.
Grapefruit Peel	Possesses potent antifungal and antibacterial properties, rich in antioxidants to build a strong immune system (fights off infections and free radicals), reduces cholesterol levels.
Jasmine	Reduces inflammation, promotes sleep and relaxation, antibacterial, and antiviral.
Lemongrass	Reduces digestive discomfort, acts as a painkiller, and reduces cholesterol levels.
Licorice	Raises blood pressure (helpful for those with chronic low blood pressure, dizziness), enhances healing of stomach ulcers, soothes sore throats.
Nettle	Eases issues associated with muscles and joints (arthritis, rheumatism, tendonitis), reduces skin conditions (including eczema), counters respiratory ailments (including asthma and coughs).
Oat Straw	Strengthens and builds bones, calms nerves, and reduces anxiety; painkiller.
Orange Peel	Possesses antifungal, antibacterial, antiviral properties, prevents growth of tumors and cancers, enhances digestion and reduces bloating.
Passion Flower	Promotes sleep and relaxation, lowers blood pressure, painkiller (especially good for menstrual pain).
Peppermint	Improves digestion and eases digestive discomfort (symptoms associated with IBS, nausea, flatulence, heartburn), painkiller, reduces congestion and coughs.
Reishi	Possesses anti-cancer properties, soothes nerves and promotes calmness, anti-aging.
Rose Petal	Strengthens the immune system, therefore helps fight infections, rids body of toxins, eases insomnia and fatigue.
Rosehip	Strengthens the stomach, reduces diarrhea, eases coughs.
Sage	Soothes mucous membranes within mouth, throat, and tonsils, aids in digestion, promotes healthy gums.
Slippery Elm	Soothes sore throats, irritated digestive tract, and skin.
Turmeric	Prevents cancer, decreases inflammation of all types, fights heart disease.
Vanilla	Eases anxiety, reduces stress, promotes relaxation, works as an aphrodisiac, enhances libido, reduces fever.

A Ribbon on Your Finger: Drink more water throughout the day with gentle reminders. Put eight rubber bands at the bottom of your eight- to ten-ounce glass, or three rubber bands on your one-liter size stainless-steel water bottle. When you finish one glass or bottle, move the band to the top. Repeat with remaining bands. Once all are at the top, you are done for the day and can move them back to the bottom and start again tomorrow.

BUT WHAT'S THE BEST WATER TO DRINK?

Many people, including myself, feel blessed to live in a place where drinking the tap water won't kill us — at least not instantly. But there is a lot in my tap water I prefer not to consume regularly, like chlorine and fluoride, to name but two. I could throw in the xenoestrogens (toxic hormone-like substances that mimic the body's own estrogens and have been implicated in breast and prostate cancer) if you want me to name three. I'm afraid that unless we call over the local water testers to check our very own tap water, we may never know the full story of what really is in the water we're drinking. Because of this uncertainty, many of us try to avoid tap water. Then there are the problems of bottled water, and where that water actually comes from, not to mention that it sits around in plastic, leaching chemicals such as BPA (see page 171), which contribute to the man-boob epidemic and all the hermaphrodite tadpoles filling our lakes.

At this point in your UnDiet journey, your primary concern is that you are drinking enough water every day. Don't be afraid of tap water. What kind of water do you think is being used in your coffee, soda, and fruit juice? One and the same, my sweet.

Only after you've got the water guzzling sorted and well established into your life should you start to concern yourself with the type you are taking in. My personal preference is spring water straight from the source. I have been known to take a whole bunch of glass bottles to a local spring to stock up. Short of harvesting fresh spring water, steam distilled or reverse osmosis are great options if you live in an urban center. Counter-top filtration systems can also be very cost effective. When I do drink filtered water, I like to add a little sea salt, lemon juice, or marine phytoplankton to help re-mineralize what's been taken out. Straight tap water is not ideal, but the worst of the worst is plastic-bottled water. It's often not much better than tap water and is made worse by sitting around in plastic for who knows how long, adding to the waste in your body and the waste on the planet. Not good.

UNDIET LIVING

UnDiet for Abundance Mantra

Chug-alug, chug-alug. Drinking my water, cleansing my cells.

Make Love in the Kitchen

All drinks are not created equal.

❀ Farewell, fruit juices (all natural and sweetened).

❀ So long, sodas (diet or regular).

❀ Adios, alcohol.

❀ Call me later, caffeine (including black tea and energy drinks).

TRANSITIONAL TIPS AND TRICKS TO MAKE IT HAPPEN

❀ **Start your day with lemon and cayenne in 8–16 ounces of water.**
This will add a super flush to your morning routine. Overnight, your body does a lot of healing and repairing that produces waste matter. Starting your day by guzzling this cell-flushing tonic will get everything moving. It will alkalinize your body, flush your cells, enhance circulation, and aid in elimination. (You can find this recipe on page 55.)

❀ **Drink that water down.**
Drink eight to ten glasses of water per day, or about 68 ounces. This is obvious at this point. It's an absolute essential. Stop sipping back the calories and start drinking your way to abundant, vibrant health.

❀ **Replace at least one coffee/black tea with an herbal alternative.**
Start off easy, replacing just one. Maybe the mug gets smaller first and then gets replaced by a more health-promoting option. Once you've mastered the one switcheroo, you can move on to two.

❀ **Get juicy.**
Green juice is a party for your cells. Add extra greens to your juices, or order a green cocktail at your local juice bar. The more greens you drink, the sweeter they will taste.

❀ **No ice, please.**
Practice saying that. Get the most hydration from your sipping by consuming your drinks at room temperature or warmer.

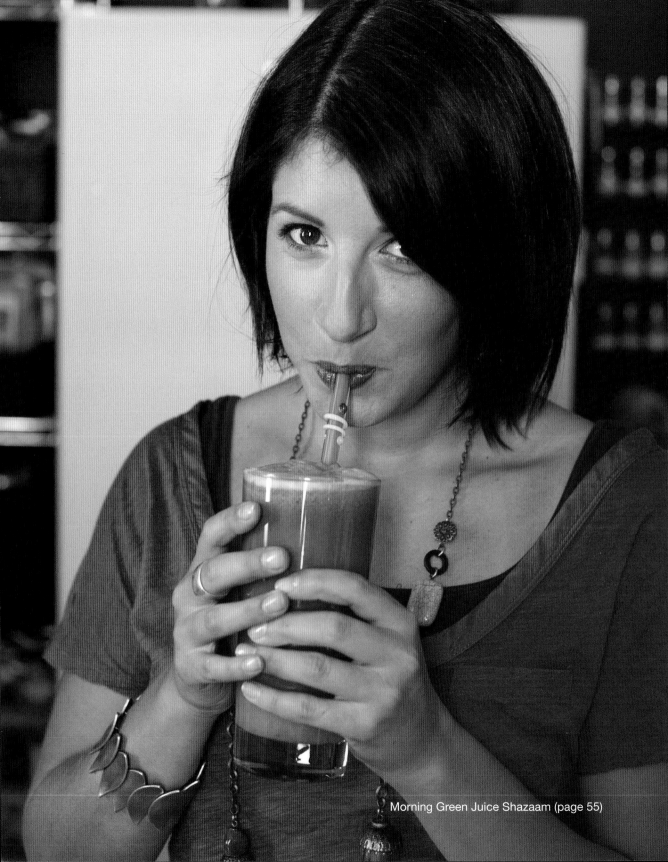

Morning Green Juice Shazaam (page 55)

Lemon, Cayenne, and Water

Serves: 1

½	lemon, juiced	½
	pinch of cayenne, or as much as you can handle	
16 oz	warm water	250 mL

DIRECTIONS

- Pour the lemon juice into a tall glass or mason jar, add cayenne.
- Fill with water and either stir with a spoon or replace mason jar lid and shake until well mixed.
- Suck that loving back. I recommend drinking it with a glass straw — easier to get down for sure!

> Lemon juice and cayenne in water first thing in the morning rehydrates the body, signals the digestive system to start working, rinses out the liver from a night of detoxing, healing, and repairing, and alkalinizes tissues to boost the immune system; an easy thing to do with massive impact.

Morning Green Juice Shazaam

Serves: 1

1	cucumber (peeled if not organic)	1
½ cup	water if using a blender	125 mL
5	stalks celery	5
1	carrot	1
3 cups	fresh spinach leaves or greens of choice	750 mL
2–3	fresh romaine leaves	2–3
1 inch	fresh ginger root (peeled if not organic)	2.5 cm
½ cup	fresh parsley	125 mL
½	apple	½
¼	lemon (peeled if not organic)	¼

JUICER DIRECTIONS

- Cut up all veggies to fit through juicer.
- Run produce through, without forcing or jamming.

IF USING BLENDER:

- Place cucumber in container, pour water overtop, and blend together.
- Add celery and blend until smooth.
- Add remaining ingredients and blend until smooth.
- Pour mix through a fine mesh strainer, nut milk bag, or cheese cloth to strain out the pulp
- Drink up as close to juicing time as you can. The sooner the better!

Freshly Blended Nut or Seed Milk

Serves: 2 to 4

1 cup	nuts and/or seeds of choice	250 mL
4 cups	water	1 L
1 tsp	vanilla extract	5 mL
1 tbsp	prepared Irish moss (optional, to thicken)	15 mL
	raw honey, coconut nectar, or maple syrup to taste	

DIRECTIONS

- Soak nuts and seeds in cold water for 2–6 hours, or overnight, then drain and rinse.
- Place nuts and seeds in blender with water and mix until smooth.
- Pour mixture through strainer or nut sack and allow milk to drain into bowl.
- Rinse blender container and return milk to it. Add remaining ingredients, and blend until smooth.
- Keep refrigerated for 3–4 days or frozen in half-quart mason jars or ice cube trays for smoothies for 2–3 months.

Get Silky Smooth

I love to add Irish moss (not to be confused with the processed, concentrated thickening agent – and digestive killer – carrageen) to my nut milks. In its whole form, it does an amazing job at making your homemade milks super thick and creamy. You can find it on many raw food websites, as well as my own – www.meghantelpner.com.

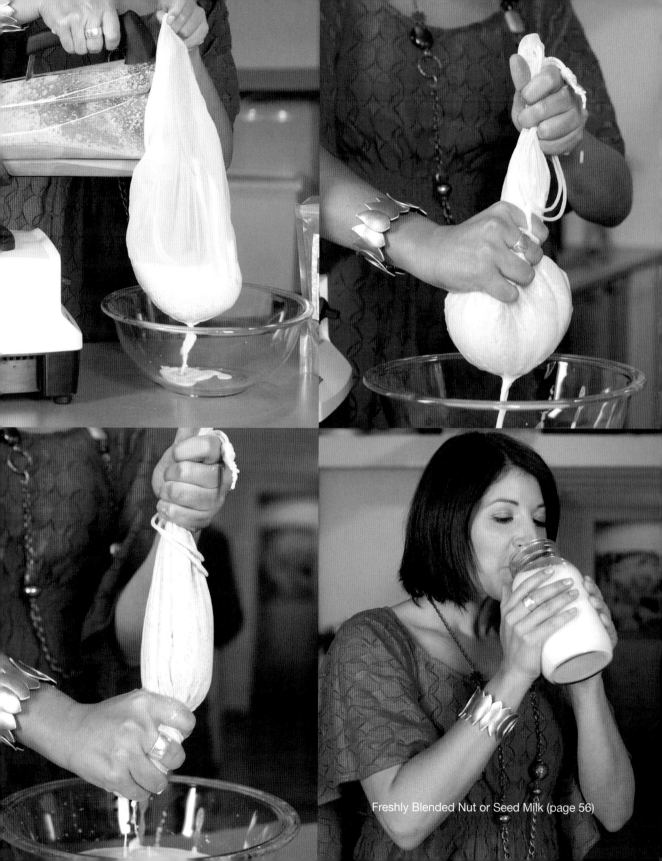

Freshly Blended Nut or Seed Milk (page 56)

Yogi Tea

Serves: 2

4 cups	water	1 L
1	cinnamon stick	1
2 tsp	cardamom seeds	10 mL
2 tsp	whole cloves	10 mL
2 tsp	corriander seeds	10 mL
2 tsp	fresh ginger root, grated	10 mL
	raw honey to taste	

DIRECTIONS

- Place all spices in a medium saucepan.
- Add water and cover, simmering for 20 minutes.
- Remove from heat and strain into mugs.
- Add raw honey to taste.

Herbal Mocha Latte

Serves: 2

3 cups	Yogi Tea or herbal tea	750 mL
½ cup	nut or seed milk	125 mL
1 tsp	vanilla extract	5 mL
1 tbsp	hemp seeds	15 mL
2–3 tbsp	unprocessed raw cocoa	30–40 mL
5	organic fair trade coffee beans	5
1 tbsp	Irish moss (optional, to thicken)	15 mL
	raw honey to taste	

DIRECTIONS

- Place tea, nut or seed milk, vanilla, hemp seeds, cocoa, coffee beans, Irish moss, and raw honey in a blender and mix. Note: If your blender has a gradual speed increase and vents steam, you can do this with warm tea. If not, blend together at a cooler temperature and then heat on the stove – otherwise the steam could cause the blender lid to burst off.
- Pour mix through strainer to remove any coffee grounds.
- Sip, sip away while writing your farewell letter to your formerly fave coffee shop.

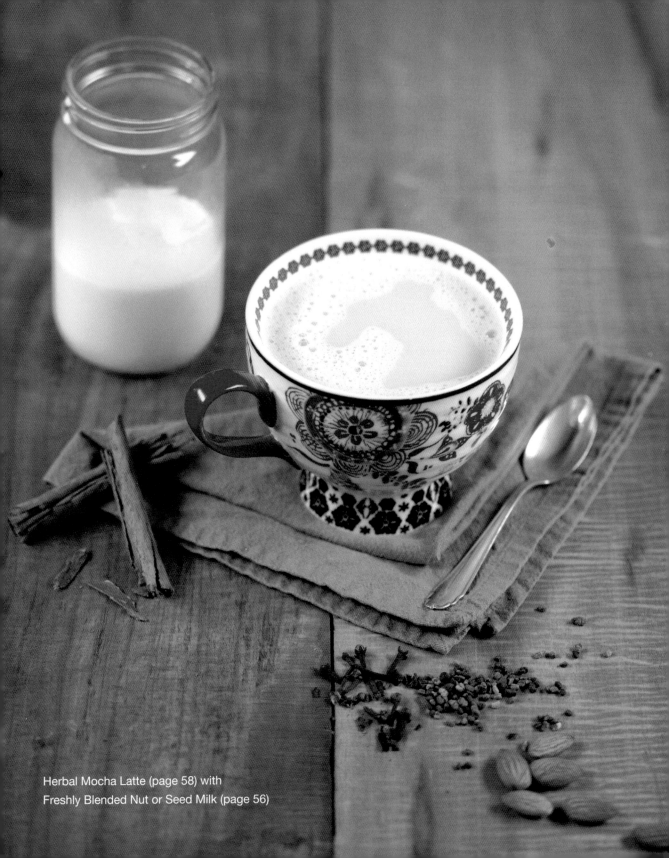

Herbal Mocha Latte (page 58) with
Freshly Blended Nut or Seed Milk (page 56)

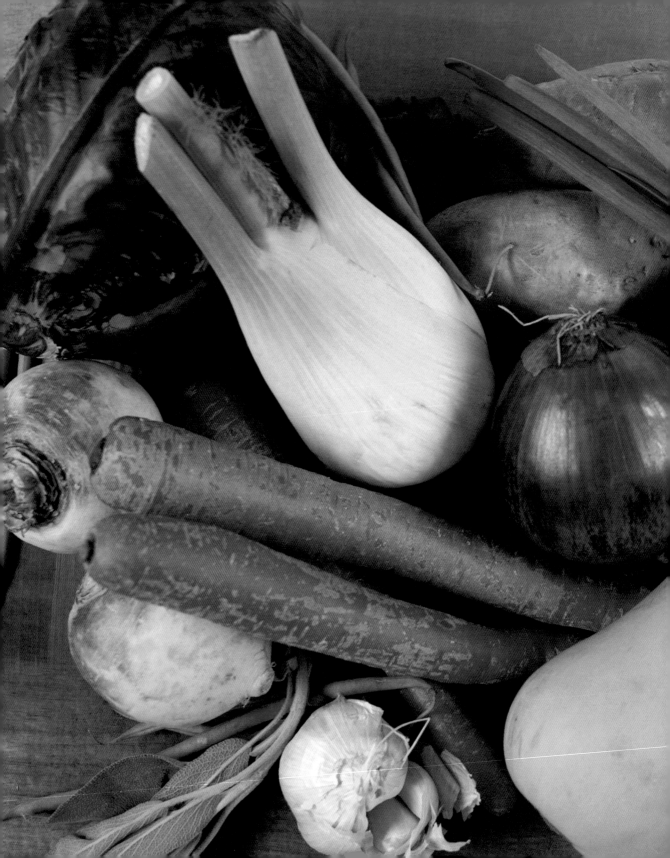

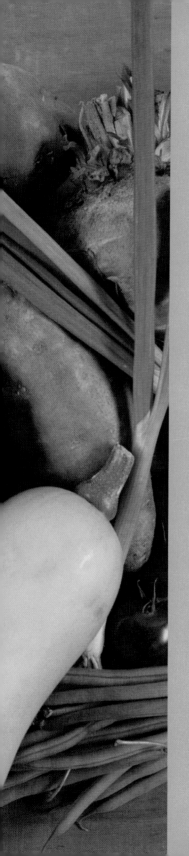

CHAPTER 4

Just Eat Real Food

One summer at the cottage, my brother Michael and my dad Ron snuck into town to pick up gummy black licorice candies. The package listed "food-grade petroleum" as one of the ingredients.

Our information resources up there are limited and I had a point to prove. In the middle of the afternoon, I went out to the fire pit and got a fire going. For their benefit, I took one of their black licorice candies, food-grade petroleum and all, and threw it in the fire. I figured anything with petroleum would have a party in the fire.

And it did. This little black licorice candy bubbled and popped and grew. It grew big. What was once a small inch-long candy grew into a four- or five-inch mass of what looked like bubbling plastic. The thing wouldn't burn, it wouldn't disintegrate, and even after the fire burnt itself out, it never turned to ash. I bet if I dug around in that fire pit, the remnants are still there years later. I can only imagine what that kind of stuff does inside our bodies.

And, no, they never ate the rest of the candies – or at least, not in front of me.

THE HEALTHWASHING OF OUR FOOD

It's a little silly-Billy that "real food" even requires an explanation, but so it goes and here is mine.

For the most part, the food we eat on a daily basis has become so complicated that it hardly resembles anything that is actually food at all. The great big giants of the processed-food biz have swooped in to try and mechanize the way we eat, as if we were little robots that worked like pre-programmed machines.

Big Food companies have genetically modified corn and soy by the city sized—farm full. This weird modern-science food-like stuff isn't even edible right off the farm. You couldn't take an ear of conventional GMO corn from a field in Iowa, peel back the husk, and take a giant chomp out of it; it would be bitter and far too fibrous, like gnawing on wood chips. What is being grown in those fields is not really food, but a wood-like substance that gets broken down into its component parts in the processing factories and then reconstituted as "food." It gets put into a fancy box with all kinds of label claims – claims I like to refer to as "healthwashing." It is flavored and sea-soned just so, making it taste perfectly delicious to our processed food–loving taste buds. The result is that we get accustomed, and often addicted to all these fakey-fake "naturally flavored" chemical products.

If everyone followed the very simple rule to just eat real food, our diets would be far simpler, far more health supportive, and contrary to popular opinion, far easier to make and enjoyable to eat. This phase of UnDieting requires us to put blinders on to food-like products that dominate magazine ads and TV commercials. We also must be careful not to fall prey to the "healthwashing" claims on packages that shout at us pro-claiming the food contained within will solve all our problems from a muffin-top belly to a slow brain, while also feeding the hungry children and supporting the "fight for the cure." A bag of processed potato chips isn't all that. It never will be.

I don't want to be your real-food guru. This UnDiet lesson is going to teach you fair and square how you can be your own real-food guru (and drop some sweet knowledge on your friends and family, too). This is not compli-cated; in fact it is actually the simplest thing in the world.

get the stories
behind the photos
http://bit.ly/UnDiet

In short, real food is about eating food in its natural, whole form. Take an apple, for example. It looks virtually the same when it comes off the tree as it does when you pick it out of your fruit bowl and bite into it. An apple is real food, as is an almond, and an egg (the kind that comes in the shell, not the white gloopy stuff that you pour from a carton).

THE DEFINITION OF REAL FOOD

Real food is pretty straightforward. It is food grown or raised with few or no chemicals, hormones, sprays, or other weird bioengineering tactics or processing — like the food you would grow in your backyard. Real food is food you recognize, that your kids should recognize, and that your great-grandmother was raised on. Real food has nothing added to it, and nothing taken away. It comes from either plants or from animals, and no part of it needs to pass through a chemistry lab before landing on your plate. Real food includes:

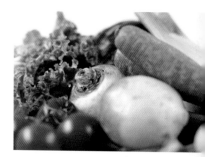

* whole grains
* beans, peas, and legumes
* fruits
* vegetables
* nuts
* seeds
* organic meat, poultry, eggs, and fish
* unprocessed dairy like raw milk and the yogurt, butter, and cheese made from it
* natural sweeteners including raw honey, maple syrup, coconut syrup, demerara sugar, black strap molasses, and date sugar
* extra virgin, cold-pressed oils including coconut, olive, flax, hemp, chia, and walnut

The Chemistry Lab and Factory Rule

For some reason we have come to think that our brains, when put together, can outsmart the eons of genius that is Mother Nature. There are many things modern science has allowed us to do — reconstruct limbs, replace organs, run machinery off sun and wind power, build cell phones — but I am not convinced that the "improvements" to our food are working.

As we UnDiet, the way the chemistry lab and factory rule works is that we will be avoiding foods that had to pass through these places. Cars? Maybe. Breakfast cereal? Not so much.

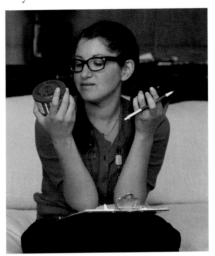

This means avoiding foods that may have been bioengineered in a Petri dish and tested to see if they could potentially harm, maim, or kill in any way. We also want to avoid foods that have to pass through a factory before they can be considered edible. This means we will be consuming foods that have rather short and very easy-to-read ingredient labels and we won't need the dictionary to decipher the contents of our afternoon snack. Perhaps most important, we will be avoiding the most notorious of villain foods: preservatives, additives, food colorings, and flavor enhancers, including the ever-popular "natural flavors."

Any food-like substance or chemical (unnatural, processed, refined and/or pharmaceutical) that we put into our body increases the toxic load we carry. A chemical that makes its home in our cells and hangs out for a while will then work toward topsy-turvying our DNA. When our cells' DNA is affected and we continue to feed ourselves disease-building processed foods, we don't have what our cells need to reverse the damage — only to perpetuate it. If our daily habits, including the foods we choose, how we handle stress, and our activity and rest levels don't work to repair DNA, improve cell-membrane integrity, and assist the efficiency of our own exit mechanism (yes — regular pooping), then we are working toward building disease. We don't want that.

SAY FAREWELL TO THESE SWEET (AND SALTY) POISONS

Artificial Sweeteners

Like white bread to the roof of your mouth, I'll stick with the declaration that artificial sweetener is poison. The definition of poison is a substance that can cause disturbance of an organism. Artificial sweeteners surely do.

As you know, what we eat will either build our health or build our disease. When it comes to artificial sweeteners, they are definitely not on the health-building side of the fence, given that they carry no nutritional benefit in terms of the presence of nutrients. Foods need to have nutrient value to hang out on that team. Often people argue that these bizarre powdery and overly sweet substances are harmless. However, all those studies attempting to prove that these chemicals are harmless have left me with a bad taste in my mouth – especially since many of these studies are funded by the companies that profit from the sales of that tested product. Here's my rule: *when in doubt, keep it out*. I prefer to avoid foods that need proof they won't cause brain and liver cancer.

The reason these sweeteners are intended for health purposes is because they are anywhere from 200 to 400 times sweeter than sugar, which means a very small amount is needed to add sweetness. This small amount doesn't register on the caloric scale or on the blood sugar meter. Calorie-free! Oh joy, oh bliss! And so people believe they are sweet and dandy and can be consumed to their heart and waistline's content. Consuming a small amount may actually be harmless, but what if this stuff ends up in your coffee, chewing gum, toothpaste, diet soda, or even some cookies, candies, or cereals a few times a week? What about every day? What about every time you brush your teeth or chew gum? What is the collective load of all that? We're no longer talking about trace amounts.

Toxins build up over time and are stored in the cells of our body, specifi-cally, the fat cells. And why do most people switch to low-calorie sweetener options? To lose weight, right? Part of the challenge with losing weight by way of consuming artificial sweetener is that, as I mentioned, they have no caloric value. However, when we taste something sweet, the brain picks up on the signal that calories/fuel/glucose (whatever you want to call it) is on the way.

The brain just got faked out by a chemical sweetener. We have momentarily satisfied a sweet craving without spiking our blood sugar or contributing to our caloric intake, but as a result of this fake out, we may find another craving soon after, as the body was all geared up for a little calorie action from food. Artificial sweeteners, therefore, can cause the poison soda sippers to either keep sipping or keep snacking with less control over intake.[1]

There is loads of really scary documentation online about the complaints filed with government health regulation boards about serious health problems associated with the consumption of artificial sweeteners. I am talking everything from chronic migraines to tinnitus (ringing in the ear), loss of vision to brain tumors. The best advice I can give is just stay away. Far, far away! Chapter 8 has some natural sweetener options to help curb those cravings.

Monosodium Glutamate (MSG)

This villain of an additive goes by many names (see page 67) and can cause anywhere from a mild to a severe neurotoxic reaction. MSG should not be consumed. Not ever. It is not a vitamin, mineral, or even a preservative, as many people assume. It does nothing but enhance the flavor of food in a very harmful way. MSG hooks us by attaching to glutamate receptors located on major organs in our body, including the pancreas and heart, and has the potential to cross the blood-brain barrier, enabling direct access to the brain. It is an "excitotoxin" or "neurotoxin," meaning toxic to the brain and nervous system and has a very harmful, degenerative effect.

MSG is produced by breaking down and changing natural-bound glutamate, an amino acid that the body produces, into free-form glutamate. These free glutamates can enter the bloodstream up to ten times faster than bound or natural glutamates, and, in these rapidly absorbed concentrations, have the ability to enter the brain via membranes in the mouth (bypassing digestion), as well as enter the bloodstream via digestion. In the past fifty or so years, MSG has become present in a massive variety of processed foods, both conventional and organic, in higher and higher concentrations.

Aside from the common headache or nausea-type side effects, MSG is contributing to our largeness as a population. One of the most consistent effects of MSG and other excitotoxins like aspartame is that they switch our metabolism to an insulin- or adrenaline-dependent mode, which in turn makes us store more fat. It is this cycle that makes us feel hungry after pigging out at an all-you-can-eat Chinese buffet (MSG poisoning is often referred to as "Chinese Food Syndrome" for its prevalence in Westernized fast-food versions of this cuisine), or why we might sit down to a handful of BBQ potato chips and soon find that we've eaten the whole bag. People eat more of a food when there is MSG in it, and we crave it when we haven't had a fix in a while. The chemical itself then causes us to feel fatigued after digestion. A cycle occurs: we eat crappy food and then lie around on the couch until we crave more of the crappy food. MSG is a bit like the nicotine of the junk-food industry.

Food Additives or Ingredients That May Contain MSG

- ❀ autolyzed yeast
- ❀ bouillon
- ❀ broth
- ❀ calcium caseinate
- ❀ corn oil
- ❀ flavor enhancer
- ❀ flavoring
- ❀ hydrolyzed oat flour
- ❀ hydrolyzed plant protein
- ❀ hydrolyzed protein
- ❀ hydrolyzed vegetable protein
- ❀ malt extract
- ❀ natural flavors
- ❀ plant protein extract
- ❀ seasoning
- ❀ sodium caseinate
- ❀ stock
- ❀ spices
- ❀ textured protein (including TVP)
- ❀ yeast extract

Butter Replacements

Does anyone find margarine delicious? Seriously? It's weird, it has a suspicious sweet taste, and it doesn't change form whether it is laying out in the sun or put in the freezer. It's almost an extension of the plastic tub it comes in. Typically, margarine is made from a variety of animal or vegetable oils, mixed with skim milk, salt, and emulsifiers. With a similar composition to butter, about 80 percent fat, 20 percent water and solids, margarine is also flavored, colored, and fortified with synthetic nutrients in an attempt to match butter's nutritional composition. Since you are now becoming a nutritional whiz, you might also notice that given the fact that margarine's

80 percent fat content matches butter's, often they'll have the same calorie count. And if margarine declares itself low in calories, then you really have to wonder what it's made of.

Typically, in the processing of margarine, whether it be the plain, old, regular margarine or the new vegetable-oil-cocktail vegan versions, the oil is pressed from seeds, purified, hydrogenated, and then fortified and colored. Whether you opt to live life on the vegan side or not, margarine should not be an option.

These oils are highly processed and most commonly genetically modified, unless specifically labeled organic. Many of them, such as cottonseed and soy, carry loads of chemicals. The high heat processing destroys any nutrients that may naturally occur like vitamin E and omega-3 essential fatty acids. To make margarine the spreadable consistency people seem to dig, the oil must be hardened. This is done by hydrogenation or bubbling hydrogen through the vegetable oil at high temperature, a process that enables it to be solid at room temperature. This is the same property that makes it perfect as frosting on cakes. When the carbon bonds are saturated with hydrogen, the product becomes a saturated hydrogenated oil.

We've all seen the "polyunsaturated oil" declaration on margarine tubs. The reality is, the processing or hydrogenation of these oils removes their flexibility, or natural liquid state, allowing the margarine to remain solid at room temperature. Through the process, any naturally occurring health benefits of the polyunsaturated fat are denatured. Because of this solidifying process, margarine usually contains some trans-fatty acids, no matter what the label says. These are the bad boys that promote inflammation in the body.

There is no problemo with the occasional dessert that contains organic margarine. There is even less wrong with a little butter. You also might love to try cold-pressed extra virgin coconut oil in your baking and olive or flax oil on your toast. Whatever you choose, just ditch the marge please.

"QUOTABLE" FOOD REPLACEMENTS

There is more to food replacements than margarine that "tastes like butter" or artificial sweetener that "tastes like sugar." We also have to watch out for other foods that may come in quotes like "mayonnaise," "cheese," and "milk."

Bypass any and all foods that come in quotes. That is a sure sign that you are about to consume something that is a fakey-fake imitation. Dairy-free and low-carb "macaroni and cheese" should raise warning flags. Go for the real deal, with top quality ingredients, or none at all.

Fake Meat

While we are on the subject of quotable foods, fake meat needs its own category. There is usually one of three reasons people choose to avoid eating animal-based foods: their health, the planet, or animal welfare. Here's the thing: eating "meat" that started out as GMO soybeans in a mono-crop field that then had to be harvested, processed, sent halfway around the world, and back to be turned into a "chicken cutlet" or "bacon," then packaged and shipped off to the health food store to be stored in the freezer is not supporting personal, environmental, or animal health.

Make a choice. If you want to consume animal-based foods, you have to choose to eat only ethically raised, antibiotic- and hormone-free. If you want to avoid animal foods altogether for whatever reason floats your boat, then also avoid processed, preserved, and chemicalized faux foods and stick with whole grains, beans, lentils, and the like. Processed food is processed food and fake meat is a no-no. A non-negotiable.

Banning the Words *Diet*, *Light*, and *Free*

When foods carry these labels, it often means that any real fat or sugar has been replaced by a chemically processed synthetic food intended to offer the same texture, or that the calories from sugar have been replaced by artificial sweeteners. As soon as a normal food becomes "diet," "light," or "free," you know it has taken a trip to the chemistry lab. My best advice: If you still wish to eat the processed food that the "diet" version is derived from, then eat the original version – just eat less of it, less often. This applies to everything from your drinks to your dairy products.

Canola, Corn, Soy, Cottonseed, and Vegetable Oils

We're going to want to avoid these, too. This guideline may seem redundant to you after reading the bit about the butter replacements, but start looking at the packages of your favorite cookies, crackers, salad dressings, packaged dips and sauces, and you may soon find that there aren't a whole lot of options in terms of what you can buy ready-made. The one exception to this guideline is if the oil is preceded with the word organic. Otherwise, you'll be putting that ranch dressing back on the shelf, picking up some organic flax, hemp, or extra virgin olive oil, and mixing your own salad dressing. By the way, have you ever wondered what vegetable produces "vegetable oil"? Me too.

THE INITIALED AND NUMBERED INGREDIENTS

BHT is my most favorite food ever! Pass a little more of that yellow #5 and I'll gladly take seconds of TBHQ and HFCS. Yes, there's a problem here. The U.S. Food and Drug Administration states clearly on its website that they use food colorings to maintain "safety and freshness."[2] Weird, right? Perhaps I should send a bag of carrots over to see how they can be improved with an injection of chemicals. Real food is not indicated by numbers, nor are ingredient names so long and tough to pronounce that they need initials for reference. If you are looking at a packaged food and can't collect the ingredients that make up that packaged food at your local supermarket, it's not food. And you can bet you're not buying a jar of caramel color or natural flavors in the baking aisle.

Top Food Additives and Preservatives to Stay Far, Far Away From[3,4]

PRESERVATIVE	USES	ASSOCIATED HEALTH EFFECTS
Benzoic acid (E210)	Used in drinks, meats, low-sugar foods, and cereals.	May temporarily inhibit digestive enzyme function and deplete glycine levels. Can cause life-threatening respiratory issues in those that suffer from asthma or allergies.
Butylated hydroxy-anisole (E320), BHA, BHT	Used in high-fat foods such as oils, butter, meats, cereals, chewing gum, beer, snacks, and baked goods, to prevent them from going rancid.	Associated with hormone disruption and development of tumors after long-term use. BHT specifically has been linked with genetic mutations. BHA/BHT may be carcinogenic to humans.

Calcium benzoate (E213)	Preservative in drinks, meats, low-sugar foods, and cereals.	May inhibit enzyme function and deplete glycine levels. Can cause life-threatening respiratory issues in those that suffer from asthma or allergies.
Calcium sulphite (E226)	Preservative in many different foods, such as burgers, biscuits, frozen foods, horseradish, etc. Also may be used in supermarkets to make old produce look fresher.	Can cause flushing, bronchial issues, low blood pressure, tingling, and anaphylactic shock. Should be avoided by those who suffer from bronchial asthma, cardiovascular problems, or emphysema.
Potassium nitrate (E249)	Preservative in meats.	May lower oxygen-carrying capacity of the blood, may form carcinogens in the body, and can be destructive to the adrenal glands.
Sodium benzoate (E211)	Preservative found in carbonated drinks, pickles, sauces, and some medicines.	May aggravate asthma and suspected to be a neurotoxin and carcinogen. Associated with fetal abnormalities. Worsens hyperactivity.
Sodium metabisulphite (E223)	Used in wine, beer, soft drinks, dried fruit, fruit drinks, vinegar, potato products, condiments, processed fruits and vegetables, fish and shellfish, deli meats, and generally most processed foods.	May provoke life-threatening asthma.
Sodium nitrite (E250)	Used to alter the color in smoked meats and fish.	Can form highly carcinogenic substances in the body with stomach acid.
Sulphur dioxide (E220)	Preservative in wine, carbonated drinks, fruit juices, dehydrated potatoes, and some dried fruits.	Associated with gastric irritation, nausea, diarrhea, asthma attacks, and skin rashes. May contribute to fetal abnormalities and DNA damage in animals.

FOOD COLORING AGENT	USES	ASSOCIATED HEALTH EFFECTS
Allura Red (E129)	Carbonated drinks, gum, snacks, sauces, preserves, soups, wine, and cider.	May worsen or induce asthma, rhinitis (including hayfever), or urticaria (hives).
Amaranth (E123)	Wine and caviar (fish roe).	May worsen or induce asthma, allergies, or hives.
Brilliant Blue (E133)	Dairy products, drinks, and candy.	Associated with hyperactivity and skin rashes, DNA damage and tumors in animals, and increased cancer risk in humans.
Carmosine (E122)	Yogurts and sweets.	Associated with DNA damage and tumors in animals and increased cancer risk in humans.
Erythrosine (E127), FD&C Red No. 3	Used to enhance color in canned fruits, confections, baked goods, dairy products, and snack foods.	Associated with increased cancer risk.
Indigo Carmine (E132)	Used to color soft drinks, desserts, candies, sauces, cosmetics, and medications.	May cause nausea, vomiting, skin rashes, breathing problems, and brain tumors. Associated with hyperactivity and skin rashes. Associated with DNA damage and tumors in animals and increased cancer risk in humans.
Ponceau 4R (E124)	Carbonated drinks, ice cream, confectionery items, desserts.	Associated with DNA damage and tumors in animals and increased cancer risk in humans. Can produce severe respiratory reactions in asthmatics.
Quinoline Yellow (E104)	Used to color soft drinks, desserts, candies, sauces, cosmetics, and medications.	Associated with increase in asthmatic symptoms, rashes, and hyperactivity. Potential carcinogen in animals: implicated in bladder and liver cancer. Potential endocrine disruptor.

Sunset Yellow (E110)	Sweets, snack foods, ice cream, yogurts, and drinks.	Associated with growth retardation and severe weight loss in animal studies. Can contribute to life-threatening respiratory issues in those that suffer from asthma or allergies. Associated with DNA damage and tumors in animals and increased cancer risk in humans.
Tartrazine (E102), FD & C Yellow No. 5	Ice cream, carbonated drinks, crackers, canned pastas, and fish sticks.	Associated with hyperactivity, asthma, skin rashes, and migraine headaches.

THE OFFERINGS OF REAL FOOD

Foods that are vibrant and alive will build bodies that are vibrant and alive. Real food, for the most part, will go bad if we let it sit too long. This is a good thing. Do you know what happens if we fuel our life with canned spaghetti that has an expiry date, yet still allows us to meet the love of our dreams, travel around the world five times, have six children, but not spoil? It means the food is dead. We are what we eat, and I don't know about you, but I don't want to be dead spaghetti.

Real food offers us the fuel to propel our lives with abundant energy. With all of its component parts intact, real food literally works to build the healthiest body possible. This means that a grain of rice should contain the husk (fiber), the germ (full of good fats and vitamin E), and the naturally occurring starch. The other option is eating a grain of rice that is white as the freshly fallen snow, devoid of the naturally occurring nutrients but jam-packed with cheap synthetic versions, with the word "enriched" stamped on the package. Don't be fooled by "enriched foods." If you've ever bought supplements before, you know the prices range greatly. You can bet that food manufacturers are not "enriching" their products with top-quality nutrients. Most likely they are being "enriched" with poor-quality, corn-derived nutrients that are not readily absorbed by the body, and are therefore largely unusable.

THE KITCHEN CUPBOARD CLEAN OUT

Before we can bring in the abundance of real food, we are going to have to make room for the fresh goodness. This means cleaning out the fridge, cupboards, and pantry. Now, I don't expect you to drop the book this minute, pull out the garbage bag, and start sweeping in broad arm strokes the contents of your cupboards into said garbage bag. There is a rhyme and reason to the process.

Get Organized

1

* Arrange your cooking appliances in a way that will encourage use. If dragging your juicer out from behind a stack of pots is keeping you from using it, then store it on your counter and just put it away when you need more space to work.
* Group your ingredients together (all flours on one shelf, all beans on another).
* Label jars and make sure they are in clear view. Avoid buying things twice.
* Avoid clutter by storing food and cookware separately.
* Note what ingredients you already have and take stock of the basics, such as spices, oils, flours, and grains.

Clean Out the Crap

2

* Give away or responsibly discard any broken or unused kitchen equipment. The less clutter in your kitchen, the happier a place it will be to hang out in.
* If a food is not health supportive, and doesn't fall into the real-food category, you don't need it around. Remember, if it is not in your house, you will not eat it.
* Responsibly dispose of (compost, donate, recycle) food and dishes that you don't believe you will ever use.
* Check expiration dates and discard foods that are past their prime.
* Vow to do better next time, which means that you will buy just what you need, and use what you buy.

Get Stocked

3

* Read through your favorite cookbooks to see commonly used ingredients.
* Can healthy substitutions be made? (For example, subbing extra virgin olive oil for canola oil, raw honey for sugar.)
* Make a list. Note what you already have (in your neatly organized pantry) and everything you need.

Make It Easy

❉ Keeping things orderly ensures you will always find what you need.

❉ Have healthy ingredients prepped and ready on hand. This helps prevents impulse take-out orders or chip-and-cracker binges.

❉ Store your food properly to ensure it will stay fresh. This helps to guarantee your meals taste great and will save you money.

❉ Keep the foods and tools you use often most accessible.

Basic guidelines on shelf life of foods:

canned foods: two to five years

cereal: six months

pasta: one year

spices: six to twelve months (store in cool, dry place)

flours: three to six months (store in cool, dry place)

grains and legumes: one year (store in cool, dry place)

dried herbs: three months for optimal flavor (store in glass)

condiments: one year

DECODING PRODUCT LABELS

Once we start bringing awareness to the foods we eat, and perhaps even more important, to the foods we no longer want to eat, the trip to the grocery store becomes a different process. You no longer need to spend time walking up and down the aisles waiting to see what packaging hollers at you the loudest. You're going to realize pretty quickly what it means to shop the perimeter of the store – or you may choose to bypass it all together and get your produce at the local market or fruit store and your staple goods at the bulk or health food store.

The lesson here, though, is that once you start looking at the labels on packaged food, you will have some questions. What does the daily value really mean? Why does it say "contains fiber" on the label, but has just one gram on the nutrition panel? What difference does it make if the calories come from

The Only Part That Counts!
The most important part of a food label is the ingredients. If it's a bunch of things you can't pronounce or "modified" this or "concentrated" that, you're in trouble.

fat or from carbohydrates? All valid questions, and the answer, according to our UnDiet rules is very simple: ignore them.

Here I decode the labyrinth of the modern nutrition panel.

Nutrition Facts

Serving Size **A**
Servings Per Container **B**

Amount Per Serving C

Calories D Calories from Fat **E**

F **% Daily Value***

Total Fat G

Saturated Fat **H**

Cholesterol I

Sodium J

Total Carbohydrate

Dietary Fiber } **K**

Sugars

Protein L

Vitamin A } **M** { Vitamin C
Calcium } { Iron

A **Serving Size:** The amount considered one serving of the product. Every other nutrient or piece of info listed on the label is based on this amount.

B **Servings Per Container:** This tells you how many servings there are in one package. Most of us don't stick to just one serving. Trickiness!

C **Amount Per Serving:** This part gives you the details about the nutrition found in the serving size. Watch out – it's not necessarily for the whole package!

D **Calories:** This is the amount of calories per serving. Remember – it's not so much how many there are, but where they come from.

E **Calories From Fat:** This is the number of calories that come from fat. It doesn't mean a whole lot as chances are if there are few calories from fat, there are likely more calories from sugar.

F **% Daily Value:** The percentage of the recommended daily amount of each nutrient in the product, based on a 2,000 calories/day diet. Daily values are set arbitrarily by government bodies and don't take everyone's individual needs into account.

G **Total Fat:** How much fat is in one serving of a product.

H **Saturated Fat, Polyunsaturated Fat, Monounsaturated Fat:** We need all three of these fats to remain healthy. Saturated fat gets a bad rap, but it gives structure to our cells and provides energy. What you want to avoid at all costs are trans fats, which are toxic.

I **Cholesterol:** This is another type of fat that has a bad reputation, and yet it plays an important role in making steroid hormones, Vitamin D, and bile for digestion. Only about 20 percent of our cholesterol comes from food; the rest we make ourselves. Only animal products have cholesterol – plants don't.

J **Sodium:** How much salt is in a serving. There is a world of difference between bleached and processed sodium and natural sea salt, which has a broad range of minerals in it.

K **Total Carbohydrate:** This explains the fiber and sugar content in a serving. Generally we want to avoid foods that are low in fiber and high in sugar, as these usually don't have much in the way of nutritional value. You can add up the grams from sugar and the grams from fiber and have it not equal the total amount of carbs. What accounts for the extra? Good question.

L **Protein:** This tells you how much protein is contained in a serving.

M **Vitamins/Minerals:** This tells you how much of a few select vitamins and minerals you are receiving from one serving. If a packaged food contains any of these, it's often of the "enriched" variety – meaning they've been loaded with synthetic versions of the nutrients, which are tough for the body to actually utilize.

BUT IT'S ORGANIC! IT MUST BE HEALTHY

This is perhaps one of the trickiest traps out there. Let's be clear right now: "organic" and "healthy" are not one and the same. "Natural," "whole," and "unprocessed" may also not be the best claims to ensure that what you are eating really is natural, whole, or unprocessed. I say this because if you are eating something that came with one of these labels, it likely was printed on the package of the now-processed food. Whole, real foods rarely come in packages with label claims.

"Consumers have to understand that the purpose of these claims is to get them to buy the product."
– Marion Nestle

For a food item to be labeled "organic" or "natural," it must adhere to standards that are set by government agencies. Other claims like "now contains plant sterols" or "good source of antioxidants" come from nowhere (or more accurately, marketing departments) and they mean little or nothing, which is why you'll find these claims on a package of Jello.

Doing the right thing gets tricky. Here's a little glossary that you need to read, understand, maybe even study and memorize, spelling-bee style. This might be the best guide of all to know if what you are eating is, in fact, what you think you are eating. As you'll see, very few of these claims actually have any regulation around them and it becomes the manufacturer's responsibility to be honest with their claims.

The Meaning of Food Labels[5,6]

❉ **Organic.** Any multi-ingredient product bearing the USDA Organic seal or Canadian Organic Standards (COS) logo usually ensures that the products contain at least 95 percent organic ingredients. The certification process is voluntary, and not every product that claims to be organic undergoes the same reviews.

❉ **Made with organic ingredients.** At least 70 percent of the ingredients must be organic, but cannot carry the USDA Organic or COS seal.

❉ **Non- or -free. Must have less than the following per serving:** fat (0.5 gram), sugar (0.5 gram), cholesterol (2 milligrams), or sodium (5 milligrams).

❉ **Low.** Generally, the product must have less than the following per serving: fat (3 grams), cholesterol (20 milligrams), or sodium (140 milligrams).

❉ **Reduced.** Generally, the product must have at least 25 percent less of the given component than is typically found in that type of food.

❉ **Light.** If at least half of the product's calories come from fat, fat must be reduced by at least 50 percent per serving. If less than half of the calories are from fat, fat must be reduced at least 50 percent, or calories reduced at least 33 percent per serving.

❉ **Reduced, added, extra, plus, fortified, or enriched.** These claims can be made relative to a similar representative product.

❉ **High, rich in, excellent source of.** All designated products with at least 20 percent of the recommended daily amount per serving.

❉ **Good source, contains, provides.** The product must have more than 10 percent but less than 20 percent of the recommended daily amount per serving.

❀ **More, fortified, enriched, added, extra, plus.** For vitamins, minerals, protein, and fiber with at least 10 percent of the recommended amount per serving.

❀ **Lean.** Generally, less than 10 grams of fat.

❀ **Extra lean.** Less than 5 grams of fat.

❀ **Certified humane.** A label for products made by non-profit organizations dedicated to humane treatment of animals. To use the label, animals must have been given no growth hormones or antibiotics, not lived in cages, crates, or stalls; and must have had "access to sufficient, clean, and nutritious feed and water."

❀ **Naturally raised.** A recent standard for animals raised without growth hormones or antibiotics.

❀ **Natural.** A term regulated only for meats and poultry, containing no artificial flavors, colors, or chemical preservatives, and otherwise meaningless.

❀ **Farmed, wild caught.** A term referring to seafood. Farmed fish are raised in captive environments, often eating carnivorous diets, and tend to be fattier as they aren't given the space to swim around. "Wild caught" refers to fish that were caught in their natural habitat and tends to be a healthier and more sustainable choice when selecting certain fish.

> *"We can make a commitment to promote vegetables and fruits and whole grains on every part of every menu. We can make portion sizes smaller and emphasize quality over quantity. And we can help create a culture – imagine this – where our kids ask for healthy options instead of resisting them."*
> *– Michelle Obama*

Then there are the labels that are mostly made up that confuse us when we're at the store. They're "healthwashing" claims:

* contains antioxidants
* doctor-recommended
* free-range (can mean anything from an animal that roams freely to one that is let out of its cage from time to time)
* green
* immunity formula
* kid-approved
* made with whole grains
* may lower cholesterol
* natural (for non-meat or -poultry products)
* natural goodness
* no trans-fat
* non-toxic
* parent-tested
* strengthens your immune system

Navigating the labels and claims on all the other stuff is really hard work — work that comes with no reward. With all the confusion that surrounds labels, ingredients, nutritional values, and what-not, I'll bet you're about ready to take up the role as head cheerleader for the Real Food Team. Ready to human pyramid and back handspring over Real Food?

"The average person is still under the aberrant delusion that food should be somebody else's responsibility until I'm ready to eat it."
– Joel Salatin

UNDIET LIVING

UnDiet for Abundance Mantra

Eat real food.

Make Love in the Kitchen

Chemicals are no longer a food group in our UnDiet.

* Avoid foods containing preservatives, additives, artificial sweeteners, and other weird chemicals.
* Avoid foods that passed through a chemistry lab or factory.
* Get the bad stuff out of your house. Cleanse the junk to make room for the healing goodness.
* Don't fall into the label claim trap.

TRANSITIONAL TIPS AND TRICKS TO MAKE IT HAPPEN

* **Read the ingredient list, not the nutrition panel.**

  Calorie counts and sugar content are irrelevant. Focus on the actual ingredients in the food you're eating. It's not a question of math and quantity; you want to focus on quality.

* **Cleanse the kitchen.**

  Make your kitchen a place you want to be. Do a big clean out every three or four months to stay on top of it and clean out the fridge every two weeks. The more pleasant the space is to be, the more you'll want to be in there.

* **Start asking questions.**

  Go on, don't be shy. Talk to your grocer, your butcher, the cheese and egg people. Go to the farmer's market and get chatting. Talk to the people selling your food and other people buying food. Find out where your food is coming from and how far it had to travel to get to you. Get to know the person who is growing, preparing, and cooking your food.

* **Shop the perimeter.**

  Think of how much time you'll save on grocery shopping! Stick to whole foods for most of what you eat – that means starting in the fruit and veggie section and loading your cart up there first.

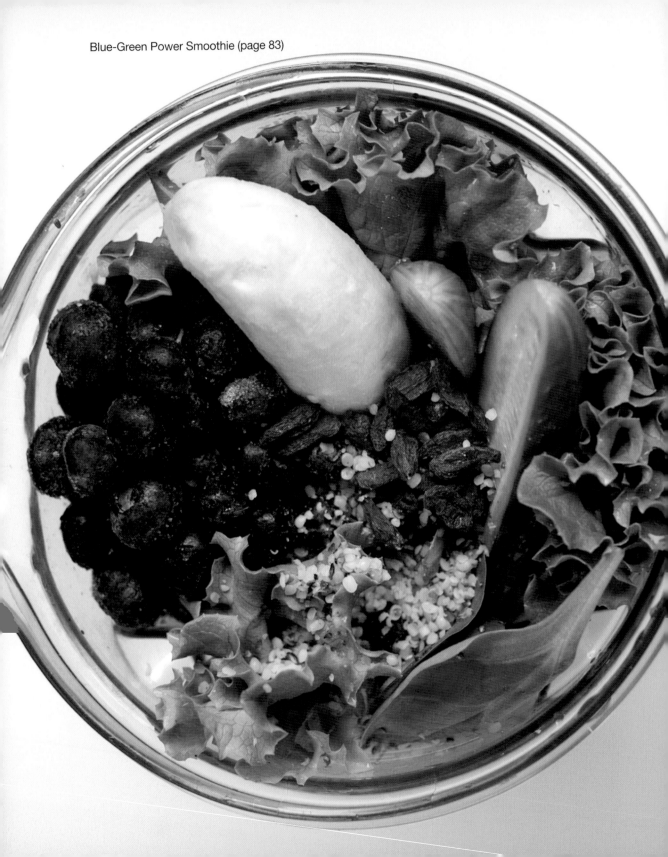

Blue-Green Power Smoothie (page 83)

Blue-Green Power Smoothie

Serves: 2

½ cup	fresh or frozen blueberries	125 mL
½	fresh or frozen banana	½
5	leaves romaine lettuce	5
1	handful baby spinach	1
4 inches	cucumber	10 cm
2 tbsp	goji berries	30 mL
2 tbsp	hemp seeds	30 mL
1 tbsp	chia seeds	15 mL
1 tbsp	coconut oil	15 mL
1 tbsp	raw honey	15 mL
1 cup	ice	250 mL
2 cups	water (more or less depending on desired consistency)	500 mL

DIRECTIONS

» Add all ingredients to blender, and process until smooth. If you don't have the best blender in the whole world, blend some of the liquid ingredients first, then add the tougher stuff.

Whole-Grain Porridge

Serves: 1

½ cup	rolled oats	125 mL
1 cup	water	250 mL
1 tsp	coconut oil	5 mL
2 tsp	cinnamon	10 mL
½	apple, cubed or grated	½
1 tbsp	ground flaxseeds	15 mL
1 tsp	maple syrup or raw honey (optional)	5 mL

DIRECTIONS

» Using a fine mesh sieve, rinse oats until water runs clear.

» Place oats, water, coconut oil, cinnamon, and apple in a pot. Bring to boil and then reduce to simmer. Cook for about 10 minutes.

» Stir in additional water until desired consistency is achieved.

» Remove from heat, stir in ground flaxseeds, and drizzle with raw honey or maple syrup.

Homemade Vegetable Stock

Serves: 8

6	large carrots peeled and cut in ½-inch / 1.25-cm pieces	6
2	parsnips peeled and cut into ½-inch / 1.25-cm pieces	2
8	celery stalks, sliced in 1-inch / 2.5-cm pieces	8
2	onions, quartered	2
1	bunch fresh dill	1
1	bunch fresh parsley	1
2	zucchinis, sliced	2
1	whole garlic bulb, cloves peeled	1
2 inches	ginger root, peeled and sliced	5 cm
8 cups	water or until pot is full	2 L
	sea salt to taste	

DIRECTIONS

- Put all ingredients into the pot, fill with water, cover, and bring to a boil.
- Lower heat and simmer for 2–8 hours. The longer you simmer the stock, the more concentrated it gets.
- Once fully cooked, allow the stock to cool for about 20 minutes, then pour through a colander.
- Transfer the quantity you want to use immediately to jars for the fridge.
- To freeze the remainder, transfer to ice-cube trays or jars, leaving about two inches at the top of the jar for expansion.

Cran-Apple Green Salad

Serves: 3–4 as a meal, 6 as a side

¼ cup	raw, unsalted sunflower seeds	50 mL
8 cups	mixed greens	2 L
½ cup	fennel bulb, thinly sliced	125 mL
1	apple, sliced in shoestring strips	1
¼ cup	dried cranberries	50 mL

HONEY-CIDER DRESSING

½ cup	extra virgin olive oil	125 mL
¼ cup	raw honey	50 mL
¼ cup	lemon juice	50 mL
2 tsp	Dijon mustard	10 mL
	sea salt to taste	

DIRECTIONS

- Using a dry pan (no oil) over medium heat, lightly toast the sunflower seeds until slightly browned and fragrant. Set aside to cool.
- Toss salad ingredients, including cooled sunflower seeds, together in large salad bowl.
- Put dressing ingredients in a mason jar, secure the lid, shake, and then drizzle over salad.

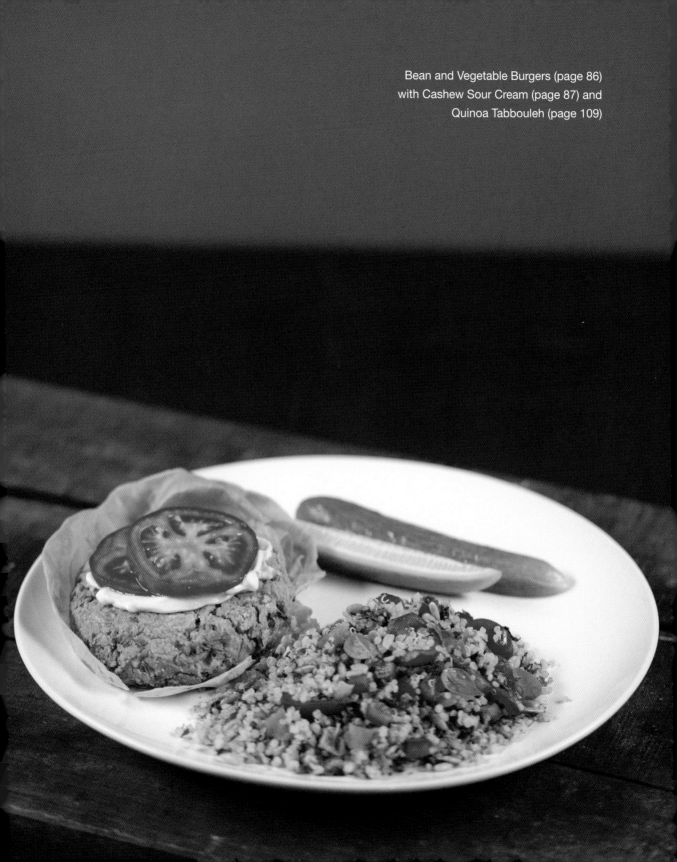

Bean and Vegetable Burgers (page 86)
with Cashew Sour Cream (page 87) and
Quinoa Tabbouleh (page 109)

Bean and Vegetable Burgers

Makes: 10 patties

15 oz	can organic chickpeas, fava, or white beans (or about 2 cups cooked)	425 g
2 tbsp	lemon juice	30 mL
1 tbsp	curry powder	15 mL
1 tsp	sea salt	5 mL
2 tbsp	exta virgin olive oil	30 mL
1	organic egg, or 1 serving of chia paste (see page 87)	1
1 cup	zucchini, coarsely grated	250 mL
1 cup	carrot, sweet potato, or butternut squash, roughly chopped	250 mL
½ cup	kale, finely chopped	125 mL
½ cup	whole-grain or bean flour	125 mL
½ tsp	baking powder	2.5 mL

DIRECTIONS

- Preheat oven to 400°F (200°C).
- Place beans, lemon juice, curry powder, sea salt, and olive oil in food processor with the S-blade and mix until smooth. Transfer mixture to a bowl.
- Stir egg or chia paste into bean puree and mix well; stir in vegetables.
- Mix in flour and baking powder. If the batter seems too wet, add more flour, 1 tbsp at a time.
- Using about ¹/₃ cup (75 mL) of the mix, form round and slightly flat patties, and place on parchment paper–lined cookie sheet.
- Bake for 25–30 minutes until slightly dry. Using a spatula, carefully flip the patties over and bake for another 5–10 minutes, or until slightly golden.
- Allow to cool for 5 minutes and serve.
  Patties will keep in the fridge for 3–4 days and in freezer for about two months in an airtight container. Just make sure they're fully cooled before you freeze them; you don't want any freezer-burn crystals forming on your creation.

Menu Staple: These burgers make fantastic toppers to a green salad, great fillers in a sandwich or wrap, and a fantastic side dish to any meat- or veggie-based meal.

Chia Paste: The Best Egg Replacement Ever

If you're of the non-egg-eating variety, have no fear. In many recipes, eggs are used simply as a binding agent and don't have any real bearing on the end result of your efforts, other than to, well, bind. Chia has a wicked gelatinous property. When ground and mixed with warm water, it forms an awesome paste that is great for replacing eggs to make baking recipes vegan, and also to replace the stickiness of gluten when using gluten-free flours.

Chia Paste Egg Substitute

1 tbsp	chia seeds, ground	15 mL
¼ cup	warm water	75 mL

DIRECTIONS

- Mix thoroughly and let sit for 10 minutes before using.

Cashew Sour Cream

Serves: 12 as sandwich spread

1 cup	raw cashews, soaked for 4–6 hours (will help it blend smoother)	250 mL
½	red bell pepper, chopped	½
2 tbsp	fresh lemon juice	30 mL
2 tbsp	extra virgin olive oil	30 mL
1 tbsp	cider vinegar	15 mL
½ cup	water	125 mL
¾ tsp	sea salt	4 mL

DIRECTIONS

- Rinse cashews, discarding the soak water.
- Place all ingredients in a blender or food processor and process until smooth.
- Pour into a glass jar and store in your fridge for up to 3 days.

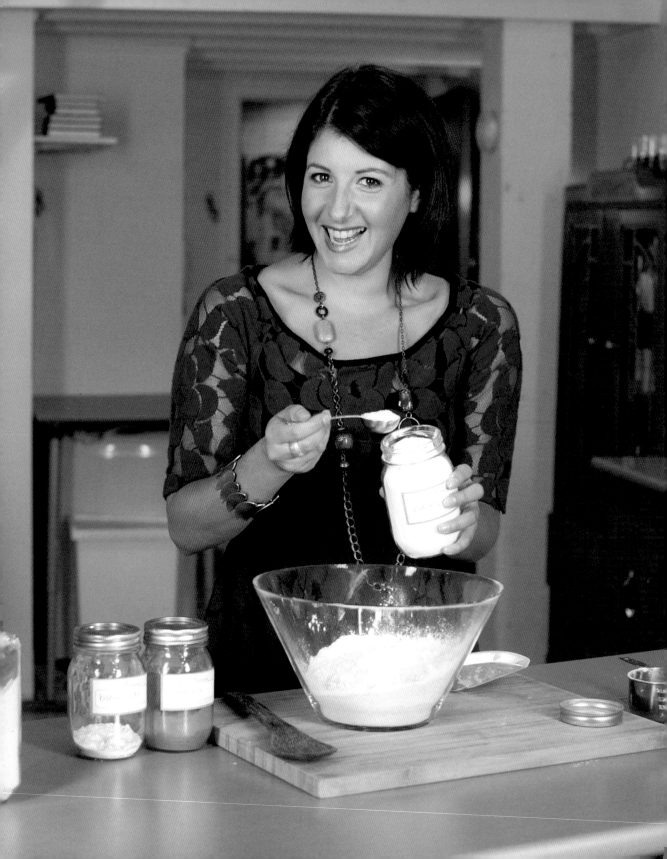

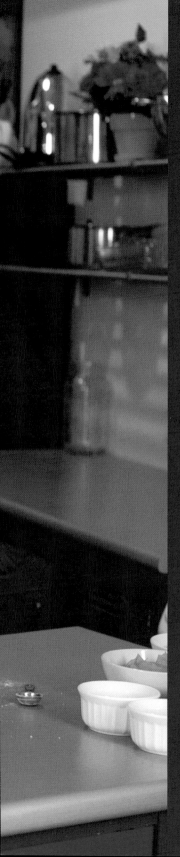

CHAPTER 5

Making Love in the Kitchen

Y ou ready? Repeat after me: *Well, hi there, kitchen! So great to see you. I know, we don't spend enough time together and when we do, I seem so rushed, even resentful that we have to be together at all. Please forgive me, for you are about to meet a new, more loving me. Time together, you and me, making a little love in the kitchen, is soon to be the highlight of my day!*

I could probably create an entire career out of cheerleading for the benefit of spending a little more time in the kitchen every day. Wait a second. I have.

Why aren't you in the kitchen cooking more? No – let me guess the reasons. In no particular order they are:

❋ not enough time;
❋ not enough money; or
❋ the ridonkulous belief that "I'm a terrible cook."

I'll address the first two by pointing out a few things. If you have a Facebook account and you have a cell phone, then you have both time and money. Do you realize that ten years ago, you likely had the very same excuses for not cooking and you didn't have a cell phone that can do everything short of scrub behind your ears for you, and Facebook didn't exist?

According to Nielsen, in 2010 the average Facebook user spent seven hours per month looking at pictures of their high-school boyfriend's wedding photos and the like.[1] (Okay, Nielsen didn't say the bit about high-school loves. I added that). That's about twenty minutes a day. You could make one kickass meal in twenty minutes with the bonus of leftovers for the next day. As well, on average, we spend fifty dollars per month on our cell phones — and that doesn't count the ones we get for our kids.

We have the time and we have the money, but for some reason we prefer to direct it to places that offer a virtual experience with instant gratification. It's the same thinking that leads us to eat donuts or drink that fourth cocktail even though we know that neither does much to offer us any benefit in the long term.

If you still insist you are a bad cook, then put your phone on hold for a month and take a cooking class. Done and done. Either way, you are about to learn how to spend as little time in the kitchen as possible while getting the greatest results. And you don't have to be great in the kitchen to be a good cook. You'll see.

All we have is right now, and right now sets the stage for later, so we'd best be laying down a solid foundation. We're going to need to stand tall and proud on that foundation for the vibrant life we have ahead.

5 REASONS TO SPEND MORE TIME IN THE KITCHEN

There are so many reasons why it's time for you to get into the kitchen. Don't you fret and don't you frown. I am by your side all the way.

1

Increased Awareness of What You Are Eating. When we cook from scratch in our own kitchen, it helps us to know for sure what is going into our body. Who wants to be loaded down with hidden sugar, sodium, and questionable fats? If I am going to eat sweet, salty, and delicious fat-containing foods, I want to know about it, and I best be enjoying it! Without the hidden villains that sneak in through food processing, we are better able to eat to our heart's content without having to bring calorie and fat-gram math into the mix.

Promote Your Commitment to Health and Well-Being. There is nothing more nourishing than a fresh-cooked meal. The ingredients themselves are at their best. Don't believe me? Come over and have a home-cooked meal with my family. Sounds fun, right? Delicious? Of course. So, why aren't you doing it for yourself?

2

Save Your Moolah for Other Fun Stuff. It is easy to go out and pick up a cheap meal, or what seems to be cheap at the time, but there are always hidden costs involved (think healthcare, sick days, and other jazz like that). If you want good food, picking up fresh ingredients will always be the most economical solution. You'll be getting more for every bite.

3

Reconnect With How Food Makes You Feel. Some meals will make us feel really great, energized, and enlivened, while other meals will drag us down, make us want to unbutton our jeans, and take a nap. When a meal is mindfully prepared and mindfully consumed, we know what we are eating, we take the time to taste the food, and we pay far more attention to how we feel when we are done.

4

Moderate Your Portion Sizes. The amount of food served at restaurants is kind of insane, with most meals big enough for two or three people. When we eat at home, our plates are usually smaller, we take what we feel we need, and we are less inclined to overeat simply because a massive portion size has been dropped in front of us.

5

OPTIMIZING YOUR TIME IN THE KITCHEN

Even though you are about to commit to spending just a sprinkling more time in the kitchen, I also know that time is tight. This is why we want to optimize that time so you can get the most done lickety-split.

I can guarantee that if you can spend an extra twenty minutes a day in your kitchen, your life might just turn out brand-shiny new and vibrant in no time. The first step is to embrace these twenty minutes not as a chore but as your time. Make your kitchen the place to be. Give it a fresh coat of paint, if that's what it needs. Get some music going in there, or perhaps what's even better for you is to shut all the doors and make it your quiet time. Get a kick-ass new knife (or get your used and abused ones sharpened), rock out the cutest apron you ever did see, and make this part of your daily UnDiet life of your dreams routine. Time in the kitchen is now a non-negotiable – like brushing your teeth or breathing.

Let's break down the many sweet-and-simple ways you can optimize your time in the kitchen.

Menu and Meal Planning

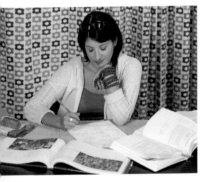

The first step to optimizing time on the kitchen clock is to actually know what you need to be doing in there. Staring into a fridge and shuffling through cupboards does not make a meal. To save time over the long run, I will introduce you to a skill our mommas learned in their high-school home economics classes: menu and meal planning, but without the canned creamed corn and meatloaf. Note, my sweet love, that this is a skill and as with all skills, practice makes perfect – or at least makes more efficient and accurate. At the very least you won't suck at it. Perfection is overrated anyway.

Use these tips to help develop a system that works for you.

Set aside the time to actually do it.
This should happen before you set aside your time in the week for grocery shopping. No one works Friday afternoon, right? This is a perfect time to look busy at work while you check your calendar for the week ahead to start the meal planning process. Give yourself an hour to start. Keep in mind that after you've done this a few times, and have a few different meal plans created, you may no longer need any time at all and you can just recycle past plans.

❋ Get a pad of paper or create a spreadsheet. Even better, download our special UnDiet meal-planning template, available on my website at http://bit.ly/UnDiet.

❉ Write Monday through Sunday across the top, and your meals and snacks down the side. Leave enough space to make any comments so you can keep notes as you go through the week on what rocked and what bit it hard.

❉ Grab any magazines or cookbooks or take a look at those recipes you've bookmarked on your favorite blogs (I hear www.meghantelpnerblog.com is a great one) for quick reference.

Note regular routines and special occasions.

❉ It can be really helpful to set certain meals for certain nights of the week and keep it consistent. For example, if you take a class on a Monday, maybe every Monday is stew/chili night, a meal that can be made in advance and frozen, or make Saturday pizza night, a great way to use up leftovers in your fridge and still have a complete delicious meal.

❉ Make note of any occasions or commitments in that week where you may be eating out, have meetings, deadlines, or events. This will affect how many meals you'll need to prepare, but can also have an impact on how much prep time you have.

What do you want to eat?

❉ It can be helpful to think in terms of categories. For example, will it be a soup and salad meal? Slow cooked? One pot? Baked? Grilled? Quick and easy (but still whole and healthy, obviously)? Try to choose different categories for different days to increase the sweet excitement of variety.

Keep it interesting.

❉ Make one or two brand-new recipes each week. When you make one you love, add that to your regular repertoire so your meals constantly evolve with your tastes and growing passion for this sweet living. And eating seasonal produce is also a good way to keep changing it up.

❉ I know this way of eating will make you smarter, but you can't remember everything. Take note of where these new recipes are located for easy reference. If it's from the Internet, create a folder online or use a bookmarking system so you know how to find it.

✿ Make sure everyone has a copy. This means keeping your meal plan accessible at home and online in the event that you need your spouse, kid, or roommate to get started on stuff or pick up some ingredients. It doesn't all have to be on your shoulders, my sweet.

Optimize the plan with creativity.

✿ Recycling isn't just for plastic and paper. Consider how certain ingredients or dishes can be repurposed. For example, a quinoa salad on Monday might mean you want to make extra quinoa to add to your soup on Tuesday and your porridge Wednesday morning. Once you're cooking something, will you want extra? A burger one night could be thrown over some greens the next day for lunch.

✿ You can't buy the whole produce aisle every time you go to the store. Pick four or five vegetables to focus on each week and use those in your recipes. Try searching online for the four or five vegetables you want to use that week, followed by the word recipe. Brilliant, right?

Make a date with leftovers.

✿ It's always nice to have leftovers of your own home cooking, and it will likely happen. Looking at your weekly schedule, there will be days toward the end of the week or on the weekend that you want to declare your day off. Make this your leftovers day (my mom calls these Fridge-Bits Meals). It's amazing what can be scavenged together with a little ingenuity and adventure.

✿ Date and label your leftovers, adding not just the date it was made but also when you think it expires. This will make sure you eat them in time!

Plan for the unplanned.

✿ Unexpected things will invariably come up. It's always wise to make a few instant meals in advance. This means having a few jars of soup, stew, or chili in the freezer and ready to go should your day become derailed and your planned kitchen time vanishes. There should be no excuse to hit the drive-thru.

✿ If by the end of the week so many unplanned events have come up that you are left with loads of leftover ingredients, why don't you:

a) cook up some soups or stews to enjoy later;

b) invite friends over for dinner; or

c) invite friends over for dinner, hand out recipes, have them help you cook and – voila! – you just had a cooking party!

SELECTING RECIPES

As you've picked up by now, I am fully shaking my pom-poms, doing round-offs and quadruple flippy-maroos as I cheer you on and build up your excitement about getting into the kitchen. This is your chance to take on the challenge, open up to the excitement, and shine brightly. Don't stress yourself out. This is going to be fun!

Before you get your tubes in a tangle, let's take a deep breath and remember that this is about easy-peasy-lemon-squeezy transitions, not stressing ourselves out and wanting to call it quits before we start. There are a few things you need to keep in mind when adding new or staple recipes to your meal plan.

Choosing the Best of the Best Recipes Ever

❋ **How much time is involved?** Most recipes have prep and cook times. These are good places to start. Choose recipes that work with the time you have in your schedule.

❋ **How many ingredients and steps are there?** Read through the recipe as if it were a riveting novel. Read the entire ingredient list and the entire set of directions from start to finish. Make sure you clearly understand the steps and know what they mean. If the list is too long (and you can decide for yourself what too long is), you'll likely put off making the dish. I typically like about eight ingredients (plus a few extra for spices) and about five or six steps tops.

❋ **Can you simplify?** I'm a big fan of recipe directions being written out step-by-step rather than as a paragraph. It may be helpful for you to rewrite the directions in a format that best suits you. If a picture is worth a thousand words for you, then seek out recipes and cookbooks that have pictures of the process, along with written directions.

❋ **Do you have the tools?** Just because you don't have the tools to make something, doesn't always mean you can't make the recipe. You may need to get creative with what you do have, or decide whether that tool is worth investing in. If you can't make the recipe work, then move on to another.

❋ **What is the cooking method?** Our goal here is to be health supportive. If a recipe calls for baking over frying, you'll want to take it. We like steaming, simmering, quick sautéing, light grilling, and baking. We take a pass at high-heat grilling, microwaving, and frying. And if the cooking method seems beyond your skill level at this point, either move along or look it up on YouTube to see if it's something you can make happen.

Make That Shopping List (and Stick to It!)

Contrary to popular belief, eating great, healthy, whole, and unprocessed food is not expensive. It may seem like it when you're at the checkout counter, but consider all the other extra purchases you make all week. Those add up, too, and likely to much more than your apples, carrots, and almonds. Eating well and healthy is not going to empty the piggy bank, as long as you stick to your list. What gets expensive is when you hit the grocery store with your list in hand, and then find yourself veering from it, filling the cart with "healthy" cookies, chips, cakes, crackers, and other treats or convenience foods. If you can make that list and stick to it, you will be amazed by the savings.

We've all had the experience where we go to the grocery store, buy the same twenty items we always buy and then come home, still without any inspiration as to how to turn those groceries into a proper meal. This is where the shopping list comes in. You've planned your menu for the week; now you have to make sure you've got the goods to see it through.

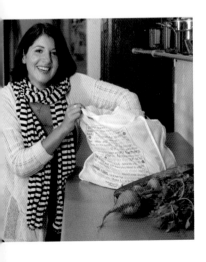

❋ **Have your shopping list nearby as you plan your menu.** I love a good spreadsheet for a shopping list. You can download a copy of my UnDiet Real Foods Shopping List at http://bit.ly/UnDiet.

❋ **Make note of everything you need.** Using my pre-made shopping list (or get crafty with your own) that has a list of all the foods you could ever want, simply highlight what is needed from the list, including how much you'll need as you go through your meal plan and recipes. If making a list from scratch, break it up into categories such as Vegetables, Fruits, Grains, Beans/Legumes, Oils, Spices, Bulk, etc. This will make it quicker in the grocery store and you'll be sure not to miss anything.

❋ **Check it twice.** Once you have your list of everything you need, go back through it, matching it up with your meal plan to make sure you haven't missed any key ingredients. The next task is to go through your fridge and pantry and check off all the items on your shopping list that you already have. You'll be left with a narrowed-down list of only the things you need. This will save you money: you're not double-buying, and you're not wasting at the end of the week. This might also be a good time to estimate your costs and stick to a budget.

❋ **Take your list with you!** I don't care how smarty-pants you think you are, you will not remember everything on that list, especially because you will now be breaking out of your usual twenty-item pattern and will be following new recipes. There is nothing more defeating than going through the trouble of choosing recipes, planning the meal plan, making the list, and then going to cook something, only to realize you missed the key ingredient. Now, the next time you do this, think of me saying "I told you so," and then make that list.

Meal Planning Magic: Jot down on your meal plan what prep needs to be done each day. Get specific here. I'm talking shapes and sizes for the dishes you want to make. This will help you to get loads done in advance and make actually preparing the meal lickety-split easy.

OPTIMAL FRUIT AND VEGETABLE PREP

When you go grocery shopping it is absolutely key that within twenty-four hours of returning from the store, you set aside twenty to thirty minutes to prep your fruits and vegetables for the week ahead. Trust me sunshine, it's worth it. I often hear complaints about throwing out vegetables at the end of the week because they didn't get eaten; prep your produce and that won't happen.

The main objective of prepping our fruits and vegetables is to make them as easy to eat as possible. This means clean them if they need to be cleaned, peel and cut them if they need peeling and cutting, and store them in the form you'll be using them in. Do what needs to be done so they will be eaten. Simple as that.

The other awesometown benefit of produce prep is that this little habit will cut down immensely on your time in the kitchen and the amount of clean up with your meals. Washing, peeling, and cutting can make a bit of a mess. Just do it all at once, and clean up all at once. Then not only are we cutting down on the amount of time needed to prep, but also on the amount of clean-up time after.

You are about ready and set to be your very own impressively prepared UnDieting Guru.

TIPS FOR EASY VEGETABLE PREPARATION

Get these things together: sink full of water for cleaning, cutting board, sharp paring knife, sharp chef's knife, and vegetable peeler.

Set Up the Vegetable-Prepping Master Station

* Turn on the radio or TV, or just zen out in silence as the master of vegetables.
* Give yourself space for the washed vegetables and have containers ready for when they're prepped. (I'm a big fan of glass mason jars and glass containers with snap-on lids.)
* Keep a bowl, green bin, or pet bunny rabbit nearby for the plant waste.

Keep in Mind How Your Vegetables Will Be Used

* If you'll be enjoying your veggies as grab-and-go snacks, cut them into grab-and-go sizes and pre-pack in airtight containers, with some water inside to keep them crisp.
* When chopping, slicing, and dicing for recipes, cut to the size indicated in the recipe and store as outlined in the chart I made for you on page 100. Before you ask, yes, there is some nutrition lost when you pre-cut your vegetables. But there is even more lost when you throw them out at the end of the week because they were too much trouble to eat.
* Save your scraps. Stalks and ends that may not look the prettiest in meals are great for cooking up soup stocks (see page 84). If you aren't ready to make a soup stock, freeze your scraps for later use.

Freeze Your Own

If a recipe calls for one cup of broccoli and you have a whole head, wash the whole thing, let dry, and freeze on a cookie sheet. Once frozen, transfer to an airtight bag or container for later use. Anything you can buy frozen, you can also freeze yourself. This works with berries, bananas, mango, winter squash, carrots, beans, cauliflower, cabbage . . . Need I go on?

No Time for Shopping? Try a CSA

If you live in the country, you likely have easier access to farm fresh goodies. In larger urban centres, there is a fantastically delicious growing movement of CSAs, or Community Supported Agriculture. This is where you buy shares in a farm at the start of the season and all through the growing season, you get your share of produce delivered to your door. If you need a more flexible option, try fresh box services where you can order on a week-by-week basis.

My Fave Shortcuts

❋ **Lemon juice:** Loads of recipes call for lemon juice. At the start of the week, juice three or four lemons and store juice in a glass jar in the fridge. Use fresh instead of bottled. Note that half a lemon is equal to about 2 tbsp of lemon juice. 1 full lemon is about a ¼ cup. This is great to have on hand for your lemon-cayenne morning drink.

❋ **Weepy onions:** No one likes chopping onions. See how many are needed for the week and chop them all at once. Store each onion in an airtight glass jar and add to recipes without tears.

❋ **Garlic fingers:** Buying garlic already peeled and minced in a jar is easy, but not so fresh. Grate up a few garlic cloves and store in an airtight jar for quick and easy fresh garlic. It will make a huge difference to the taste of your recipes. You can do the same with ginger, too.

Eat the Peel: The outer peel of root vegetables will have the highest concentration of nutrients. Whenever you have organic root vegetables, scrub the outside and enjoy without peeling. If you've got non-organic fruits and veggies on your hands, you don't want what resides on the outer layer, so your best bet is to peel them.

STORING PRODUCE FOR SUPER FRESHNESS

FRUITS	STORAGE	FREEZER FRIENDLY?
Apples	Loosely in the fridge (ditch the plastic bag). If washing first, dry before storage.	Yes. Cut into pieces, lightly toss in lemon juice, or blend into puree.
Avocados	At room temperature. Once ripe, transfer to fridge.	No.
Bananas	At room temperature.	Yes. Remove the brown peel first.
Berries (blueberry, raspberry, strawberry, etc.)	Airtight container in the fridge, with a towel to absorb extra moisture. Be sure to remove any soft or moldy berries. Wash just before eating.	Yes. Wash, dry, freeze on a cookie sheet, then transfer to airtight container or bag.
Citrus fruits (oranges, lemons, limes, grapefruit)	In the fridge.	Yes. Juice these fruits and freeze the liquid in small jars or ice-cube trays for easy use in recipes.
Grapes	Wash and dry before storing in the fridge. Remove any soft or moldy grapes.	Yes. Remove from stem, freeze on a cookie sheet, then transfer to airtight container or bag.
Melons	At room temperature and eat quickly once ripe. Store cut melons in the fridge with seeds intact, or cut into pieces in an airtight container. Consume within two days.	Yes. Cut into cubes, freeze on a cookie sheet, then transfer to airtight container or bag.
Pears	Ripen at room temperature, then transfer to fridge.	Yes. Cut into pieces, lightly toss in lemon juice, or blend into puree.
Stone fruit (peaches, plums, apricots, nectarines, etc.)	At room temperature until ripe, then transfer to fridge.	Yes. Cut into cubes, freeze on a cookie sheet, then transfer to airtight container or bag.
Tomatoes	At room temperature. Ripe tomatoes will keep for up to three days.	Yes. Puree and pour into small jars or ice-cube trays for use in soups and stews.
VEGETABLES	STORAGE	FREEZER FRIENDLY?
Asparagus	Trim ends and store in a vase or jar of water in the fridge.	Yes. Wash and dry first. Can be used in soups and stews. Not ideal for steaming.
Green beans	Airtight container in the fridge. Wash just before using.	Yes. Wash, dry, trim ends or cut into pieces.

Broccoli, Brussels sprouts, and cauliflower	Airtight container in the fridge, wash just before using.	Yes. Wash, dry, and cut to size.
Carrots	Remove tops, as they draw out moisture. Cut to size and store in bowl of water. Change water every 3–4 days.	Yes. Wash, dry, cut to size.
Celery	Cut to size and store in bowl of water. Change water every 3–4 days.	Yes. Freeze ends or small pieces for soup stocks.
Cucumber and zucchini	In crisper. Moisture will cause spoilage.	No.
Corn	Whole corn should be stored in husks in the crisper.	Yes. Cut corn off the cob and freeze the kernels.
Eggplant	Airtight in warmer part of the fridge.	No.
Lettuce, greens, and fresh herbs	First soak in cold water. Store in the fridge in a water-draining container. Do not spin until ready to use, as this will damage the cell wall and cause it to go off faster.	Yes. Fresh herbs freeze well and preserve flavor.
Mushrooms	Store in the fridge in a paper bag inside a plastic bag or large container, allowing mushrooms to breathe without drying out. Clean by scrubbing with a damp towel.	Yes. Wipe clean and freeze for soups and stews.
Onions and garlic	At room temperature in a cool, dark place with good air circulation. Can be cut to size and stored in an airtight container in the fridge for 3–4 days.	No. Freshness and flavor will decrease.
Peas	In crisper or coldest part of your fridge.	Yes. Store in an airtight bag or container.
Peppers	In warmer parts of the fridge: towards the door and out of the produce bins, which tend to be cooler. Can be cut to size and stored in an airtight container in the fridge for 3–4 days.	Yes. Wash, dry, and cut to size.
Root vegetables (beets, celery root, yams, parsnips, sweet potatoes, radishes, sunchokes, turnips, potatoes)	At room temperature in a cool, dark place with good air circulation. Can be cut to size and stored in an airtight container in the fridge for 3–4 days.	Yes. Wash, dry, and cut to size.
Winter squash (butternut, acorn, pumpkin)	At room temperature in cool, dark place with good air circulation. Can be cut to size and stored in an airtight container in the fridge for 3–4 days.	Yes. Wash, dry, and cut to size.

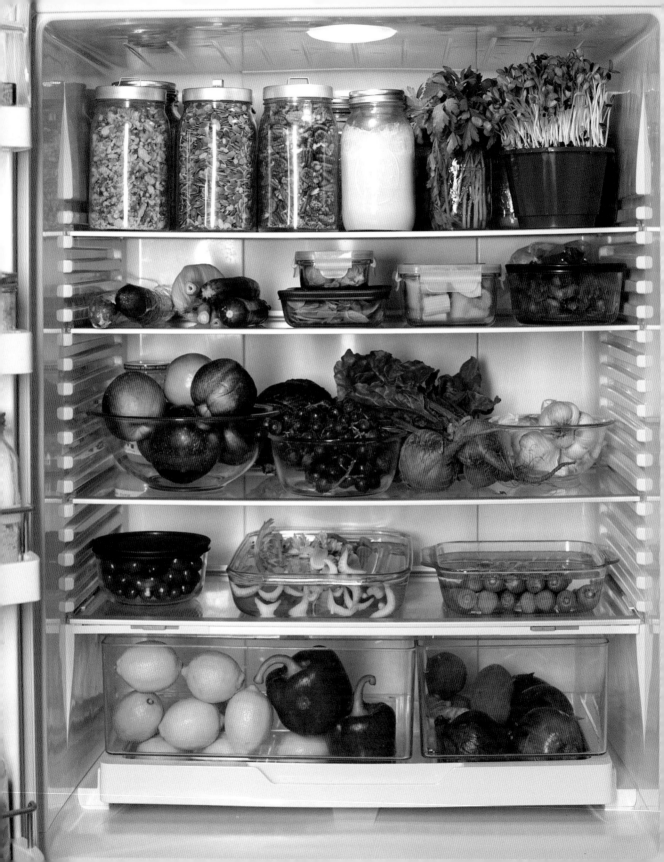

With your meal plan set and your shopping list made, you are on board to prep and properly store all your fresh produce, and we are ready to redefine what a convenience meal is.

Allow me to paint you a picture. This will be like one of those choose-your-own-adventure books that we read in elementary school.

You finish work. It is 6:00 p.m. and you are starving, tired, and you have hungry mouths to feed at home, one of them, of course being yours. You get into your car and you are torn. Do you stop by your local drive-thru joint because that seems the easier thing (Option A)? Or do you go home and get into the kitchen (Option B)?

If You Choose Option A . . . You drive through traffic, hand over your hard-earned cashola at the drive-thru, and feel a little guilty all the way home. You sit down at the table, inhale your meal, and then collapse together on the couch like a family of vegetables. (Kind of like the ones you left sitting in your fridge.)

You don't have much energy to pack lunches for the next day, or prep for breakfast. Before bed you get cravings for sweets, so you rummage around in the cupboards until you find cookies, and inhale three.

You make your way to the bathroom to brush your teeth. You have a disrupted sleep due to indigestion and the adrenaline roller coaster that has your mind spinning at four in the morning.

You wake up feeling blah, and wait until the last moment to get out of bed, leaving you rushing around without time for a proper breakfast and your family feeling the stress, too. Emotions erupt just as everyone heads out for their day, and you rush off to work feeling exhausted.

If You Choose Option B . . . You come home, the family is hungry, and everyone is waiting on you. You hop into the kitchen and dish out tasks.

You consult your meal plan. While people are tearing lettuce, setting the table, munching on the veggies you have ready to go in the fridge, and filling glasses with water, you grab a few handfuls of prepped veggies to steam and a few of your homemade frozen (veggie) burgers come out of the freezer and into the oven. You catch up with your family about their day, and spend some time together.

In fewer than thirty minutes, you have a fresh dinner that your family enjoys together. Afterward, while everyone helps clean up, leftovers are being put into containers for tomorrow's lunches, and you are getting some grains soaking or filling your blender container with your smoothie ingredients for breakfast.

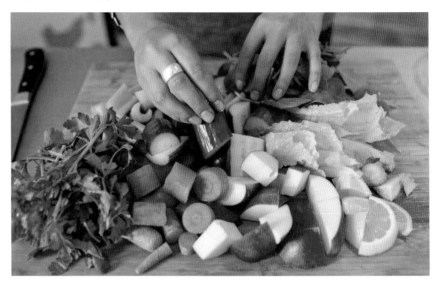

READY TO MAKE IT HAPPEN?

This transition requires the breaking of some bad habits that will inevitably lead to a lifetime of UnDieted health. You are redefining what convenience eating is and can feel great that everyone's health, including your own, will be improved because of it. We are some lucky ducks to be living where we're living with the luxury that most people in the world don't have: the luxury of being able to choose what we want to eat. Why on earth, then, would we choose less than the very best that we can for ourselves? Go on and have a think about that one.

"You can't expect to live a vibrant life when you live on Twinkie consciousness.
Not only does what you put into your mouth affect you, but it also affects the planet.
Health is a practice and honoring your body is key."
– Kris Carr

UNDIET LIVING

UnDiet for Abundance Mantra

Here I am, kitchen, and I love you!

Make Love in the Kitchen

Redefining convenience food.

* Change your thoughts around cooking. Too busy, too expensive, and skill level are excuses being left behind.
* Recycle those takeaway menus you have lying around. They are no longer your go-to.
* Frozen dinners are a no-go unless they are of your own making.
* Make space in your fridge for your easy-to-eat, pre-prepped vegetables.
* So long to spontaneous hunger-driven junk-food purchases. If it's not on your list, it's not in the cart.

TRANSITIONAL TIPS AND TRICKS TO MAKE IT HAPPEN

* **Create a menu for the week.**
  You are now fully equipped with all the info you need to create a meal plan for your week. Make the time and make it happen.
* **Plan your time to make your list for grocery shopping.**
  You can't eat fresh food without fresh food in the house. Make your list, take it with you, and buy fresh. If the grocery store is not an option or you don't have time, consider online grocery shopping and a delivery service, or your local CSA or fresh box service. It is that important!
* **Prep veggies when they're fresh.**
  Make the time, either right when you get home from the store or within twenty-four hours, to prep and properly store all your produce. It will save you time, money, and waste as you stop throwing out rotten veggies.
* **Brown bag your lunch two to three days a week minimum.**
  Since you'll be making dinner fresh most nights, you should also have fresh leftovers most days. Get creative with your leftovers and save your moolah for fun nights out, massages, and other treats, instead of a stale-bread sandwich with processed meat and questionable mayo from the lunch place around the corner from your work.

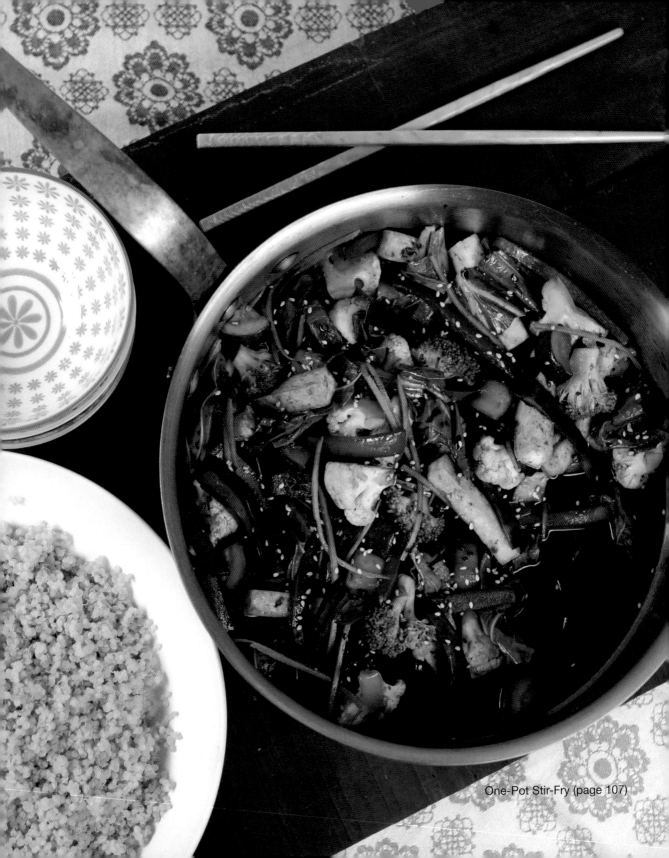

One-Pot Stir-Fry (page 107)

One-Pot Stir-Fry

Serves: 4 as a meal, 6 as a side

2 tbsp	extra virgin olive oil	30 mL
2 tbsp	water, as needed, to avoid sticking	30 mL
1 tbsp	turmeric	15 mL
3	garlic cloves, minced	3
2 inches	ginger root, peeled and minced	5 cm
½ cup	red pepper, sliced	125 mL
½ cup	carrot, grated or thinly peeled	125 mL
½ cup	each of coarsely chopped broccoli florets, broccoli stems, cauliflower, purple cabbage, and zucchini	125 mL
2 tbsp	sesame oil	30 mL
2 tbsp	raw honey	30 mL
3 tbsp	tamari (or to taste)	45 mL
4	organic eggs or ½ block of firm organic tofu, cubed	4
3 cups	collards or greens of choice	750 mL
2 cups	leftover grains (optional)	500 mL
	sea salt and cayenne to taste	

DIRECTIONS

- In a large skillet on medium, heat oil and a little water, and add turmeric, garlic, and ginger. Let cook for 1 minute or until fragrant.
- Add all vegetables except leafy greens and stir. Add sesame oil, raw honey, and tamari, and sauté for 8 minutes, until the veggies are vibrant.
- Push veggies to the edge of the frying pan and pour eggs into the middle opening. Allow to cook undisturbed for about 2 minutes. Mix together. If using tofu, add to pan, stir into the mix, and let cook for 3–4 minutes.
- Add greens and let them wilt in the heat.
- Add sea salt and cayenne to taste.
- Serve vegetable mixture on top of grains or mixed greens.

Bite-Size Bites: With any stir-fry or mixed-grain salad, try to cut all your veggies about the same size so they cook evenly. Watch out for when ingredients are added in with one-pot meals; some are added later, depending on cooking time.

Lemon Lentil Vegetable Soup

Serves: 8

¾ cup	red lentils, soaked	175 mL
¾ cup	green lentils, soaked	175 mL
2 tbsp	extra virgin olive oil	30 mL
1	small onion, chopped	1
3	carrots, chopped	3
4	celery stalks, sliced	4
1 cup	broccoli, sliced	250 mL
3 tbsp	lemon juice	45 mL
6 cups	water	1.5 L
3 cups	kale or spinach, sliced into small strips	750 mL
¼ cup	Italian parsley	50 mL
	sea salt and cayenne to taste	

DIRECTIONS

- Rinse lentils in strainer until water runs clear.
- In a large saucepan, heat oil and lightly sauté onion until translucent (about 5 minutes).
- Add lentils, carrots, celery, broccoli, lemon juice, and water. Bring to a boil, reduce heat and simmer for 20 minutes.
- Remove from heat and stir in parsley and kale. Cover for 10 minutes to soften the greens.
- Serve as is, or you can puree for a full creamy soup experience.

Quinoa Tabbouleh

Serves: 6 as a light meal, 8 as a side

1 cup	quinoa, soaked	250 mL
1½ cups	water	375 mL
1	bunch cilantro, finely chopped	1
1	bunch parsley, finely chopped	1
¼ cup	basil, finely chopped	50 mL
2 cups	cherry tomatoes, quartered and seeded	500 mL
1	red bell pepper, chopped	1
½ cup	dried apricots, chopped	125 mL
⅓ cup	lemon juice	75 mL
⅓ cup	extra virgin olive oil	75 mL
¼ cup	unsalted sunflower seeds	50 mL
1	handful of sprouts (optional)	1
	sea salt to taste	

DIRECTIONS

- Rinse quinoa in strainer under running water. Massage with fingers until it stops making soapy looking bubbles and water runs clear.
- Add to saucepan of water and bring to a boil. Reduce heat and simmer, covered, for 15 minutes or until all the water is absorbed and the grain is soft. Remove from heat and let cool, uncovered, for 10 minutes.
- While the quinoa is cooking, in a large mixing bowl combine parsley, cilantro, basil, tomatoes, and bell pepper, and apricots. Add lemon juice and olive oil and mix.
- Add the quinoa and the remaining ingredients to the bowl. Stir and serve at room temperature.

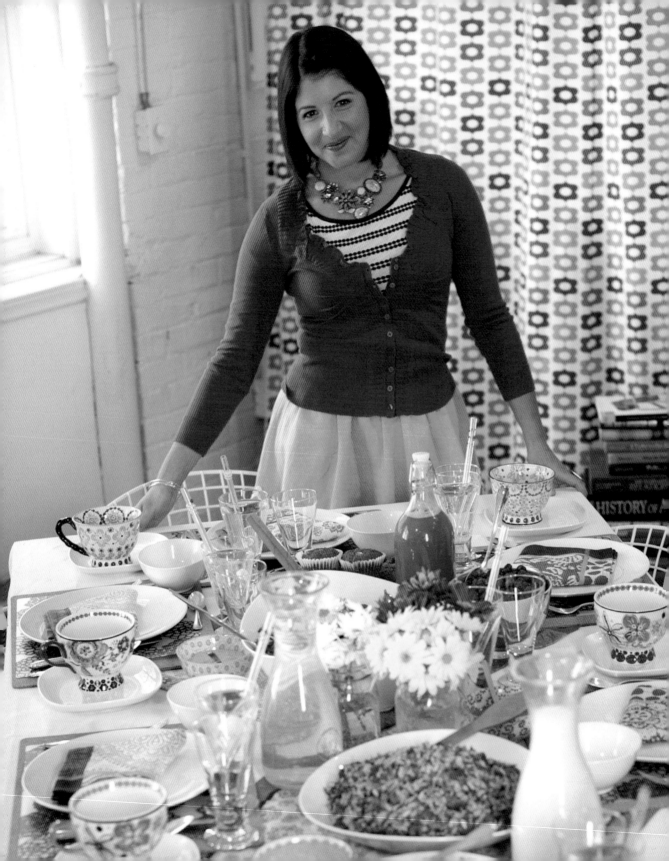

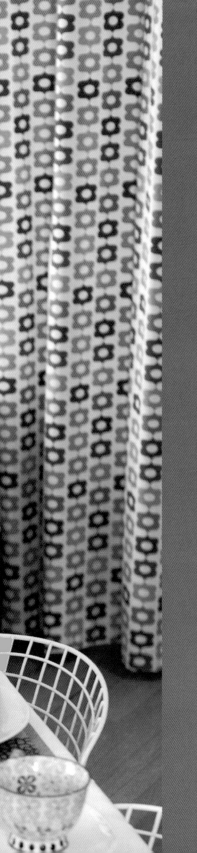

CHAPTER 6

Raised in a Barn?

A LESSON IN MODERN REAL-FOOD DINING ETIQUETTE

You want to skip this chapter. I can feel it. Don't you dare. You probably think you don't have time. You think you already know what I'm going to say. You think there will be no great nuggets of knowledge here that you can share with your friends and lovers. Well, you may be right, but then let me ask you this: When was the last time you sat down to dinner, by yourself, at a table, with cutlery, and ate a meal in silence?

Right, then. Carry on reading.

I have poor table manners. But my manners are not as poor as the boy who I dated when I was eighteen, who refused to use a napkin and would instead wipe his mouth on the tablecloth. To be honest, it was hard to reprimand him; I was just excited to be dating a guy who took me to restaurants that had tablecloths.

My own poor table manners are more of the ambidextrous variety. I eat with the wrong hands for a right-handed person, with the knife in my left and fork in the right, and I fully and completely blame my parents. It is because of this inability to hold cutlery properly that I cannot set the table correctly. Does the fork go on the left or right side of the plate? Does the spoon chill with the knife or fork, or does the spoon sit on its own at the top of the place setting? Where does the napkin go? And the glass? What if there are two glasses? Or two forks? Or two knives? Or two spoons?

Setting a table can get confusing, likely because we don't usually do it. I see it all the time in my classes. We cook up a big feast, put all the food out on the table on large platters and when it comes time to set the table, we're lost.

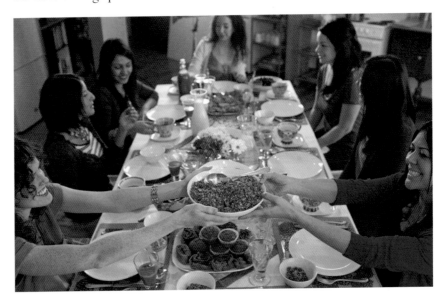

meet the ladies who lunch! bios at http://bit.ly/UnDiet

Is this because we no longer sit at the table when we eat? These days we seem to eat almost anywhere but at the table: in front of the TV, at the computer, on the phone, at our desk, in the car, in meetings. Is it possible that the change in our overall health might possibly have something to do, not just with the foods we choose to eat, but the way we eat them? I understand that there are days when time gets crunched, but if we always curb our eating habits to fit into crunched time, we will never open up that schedule to allow time for proper meals. We let the time-crunched meal become a nasty habit that leads us to eating horrid meal replacement bars and shakes that fit the recommended calorie count of a meal but not much else. A meal does not come in cellophane or a plastic tub. There are no exceptions to this rule.

By golly me, let me slip on my white gloves, and – hoity-toity, pip-pip faux–English accent – pour you a cup of tea, and offer you a little insight into the astounding health benefits of proper meal-time etiquette.

THE VALUE OF DINING AT A DINING TABLE

Beyond the fact that eating at a table with the appropriate dishes, cutlery, and napkins is one of the things that makes us the fine, two-legged creatures that we are, traditionally families eat meals together. In lands not that far away, it is still customary for a family to come home and eat the midday meal together, and dinner as a family is a non-negotiable.

A study on family eating patterns published in 2005 by the National Center on Addiction and Substance Abuse (CASA) at Columbia University found that the more a family dines together, the better the quality of relationships between family members.[1] Alternately, the less often a family eats together, the worse the experience becomes, with a decline in healthy goodness in the food and an increase in more superficial conversations.[2] A family that only spends time together when shuttling from one activity to another, and whose mealtime is drowned out by the TV, tends not to engage with each other on a particularly deep level. What may not be a huge surprise, then, is that according to a 2006 *Time* article, among families that eat together three or fewer times a week, 45 percent say the TV is on during meals, and nearly one-third say there isn't much conversation.[3]

The less we dine with others, the less we value the practice when we are on our own. That doesn't bode well for us or our wee little ones. If this is the family dining experience so many of us were raised with, it's no wonder that the evening news, the new hit show, or our iPad has become our dining companion of choice when we're on our own and often also with others.

In that same *Time* article, anthropologist Robin Fox states that "[m]aking food is a sacred event. It's so absolutely central – far more central than sex. You can keep a population going by having sex once a year, but you have to eat three times a day."[4] As food is so readily available to us everywhere we turn, it seems okay then to eat it whenever we want. There has been a shift where eating is this inconvenient thing we need to squeeze into our day so if we can refuel with a burrito while we refuel our car with gas, well, perfecto. A car can be replaced; your bod is yours for life. Take care of it.

Beyond the socialization component, there are real and tangible health benefits to dining at a leisurely pace with peeps you know and love. You will benefit not just by the über-fun social aspect, but your body will rock on a physiological level. You will literally feel better in mood and in physical body.

REST TO DIGEST

Did you know that our nervous system has two parts: somatic and autonomic? The somatic is the peripheral part that is associated with voluntary control, such as moving your arm or turning your head. We also have the autonomic nervous system that takes care of the involuntary vital functions, such as breathing, keeping the heart beating, digestion, and elimination. For the purposes of understanding digestion, understanding the autonomic nervous system is of prime importance. Ready for science class?

The autonomic nervous system is divided into two branches: the sympathetic and the parasympathetic. They serve two very different roles, both important to our survival.

Biological Effects of Being in Fight-or-Flight Mode

The sympathetic nervous system developed long ago when we lived in caves — you know, the lifestyle that often found us in the unfortunate situation of having to run from bears and tigers and what not. This is called our fight-or-flight mode, and when we are stressed blood diverts from our digestive tract and moves into our outer extremities, dilates our pupils, speeds up our heart rate, and enables us to lift a car off a trapped person in one fell swoop of an adrenaline rush. The problem is that, for the most part, we don't have to run from bears these days. This function of our nervous system is now being stimulated on a daily basis by day-to-day stresses such as getting an unwanted e-mail or phone call, being cut off on the highway, or watching intense action movies.

The sudden flood of stress hormones such as epinephrine, norepinephrine, and dozens of others do all kinds of crazy to the functioning of our body. Some of the short term, acute effects of these hormones include:

❋ Heart rate and blood pressure increases.

❋ Pupils dilate to take in as much light as possible.

❋ Veins constrict to send more blood to major muscle groups.

❋ Blood sugar levels increase to prepare for attack.

❋ Muscles tense from release of adrenaline and glucose.

❋ Smooth muscles relax – the large intestine is a smooth muscle, which is why stress can sometimes cause rapid evacuation for people (a nice way of saying diarrhea if you missed that).

❋ Digestion and immune systems shut down to allow more energy for emergency functions – yes, this is why stress results in belly gurgles and usually ends with a cold or flu.

❋ Attention becomes focused on big-picture, life-threatening attacks rather than small tasks.

Biological Effects of Being in Rest-to-Digest Mode

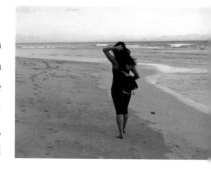

Alternatively, our parasympathetic nervous system is what we tap into when we do yoga, or go for a walk, or get into bed with lavender on our pillow, a sleep mask over our eyes, and a gentle belly massage from our partner before drifting off for a sound sleep. This is called the rest-to-digest mode: when repair and recovery happens within our body, when blood is free to circulate, when the heart rate and breathing slow, and when it is ideal for us to eat and digest our food.

The rest-to-digest, or parasympathetic mode, is the state we need to be in for healing and repairing to occur in the body.

The effects of being in this relaxed state include:

❋ Increased secretion of digestive juices to break down food and absorb nutrients.

❋ Boost in intestinal motility to get that poop pooping.

❋ Enhanced immune response, increasing our resistance to infection.

❋ Feeling of calmness, contributing to internal rest and recuperation.

❋ Increased circulation to non-vital organs such as the skin (and for men, the most prized extremity) – this increases libido and performance and gives us that sweet, healthy, natural glow.

Show Me Your Lungs: No matter where you're eating or who with, before taking a bite of food, always take three very deep breaths, expanding your belly. This helps shift your mind and body into a rest-to-digest mode, so that you can happily eat your lunch, and have your lunch do what it's supposed to do for you.

❁ Increased release of endorphins, the "feel-good" hormones.

❁ Slowed heart rate.

❁ Lowered blood pressure.

How are you feeling when you are weaving your way through traffic, watching the latest war on the news, responding to client e-mails, or even dining with a person you can't stand? If you're stressed or upset, the energy of your body is not going toward your digestive system, let alone allowing you to pay attention to what you are eating or how quickly you're inhaling it.

Eating in a state of stress is incredibly challenging to the digestive system, as chances are good your food will keep moving through you, not fully digested, leading to upset stomach and other digestive disturbances such as heart burn, reflux, and irritable bowel syndrome.

PRACTICE A LITTLE CONSCIOUS EATING

Though the concept of "conscious eating" might sound a little New Agey to you, stick with me; it may be the most important thing to learn if you really want to shift your life to the ultimate UnDiet party. Conscious eating, or eating with awareness, is about creating an awesomely positive relationship with food. Easier said than done, I know, given the truckloads of baggage we inherited from our mothers, grandmothers, aunts, sisters, and the media about diets and body image. The catch, though, is that we can't be healthy by eating the right food until we have a rock-solid, diamond-on-the-finger-worthy commitment to a positive relationship with food itself. Conscious eating is how we can start to cultivate that.

If we can take a moment here and get a little touchy feely by acknowledging that unhealthy eating patterns are often our reaction to stress, fear, and negative emotions, then we can start to make it right. See, people reach for food and will often acknowledge that it's emotional eating, claiming it brings them comfort. But being overweight and sick never made anyone comfortable. So pack up that baggage and send it off with a one-way ticket.

If we dig a little deeper into the icky prickly of it, sadness, depression, anxiety, tension, and stress drain us of vital energy. Food gives us energy. The easy answer becomes reaching for cake and ice cream to help give ourselves that easy pick-up. The challenge with our unconscious, emotionally driven food decisions is that we'll often reach for the wrong types of foods, foods that actually drain our body of energy. By eating that crap, we expend more energy than we can gain and this low-energy wheel begins (or continues) spinning. And we're that hamster running inside it, thinking it might actually get us somewhere.

Make Conscious Eating Easy

✽ Make healthy and wise food choices before you get hungry, so you aren't tempted by convenience.

✽ Choose foods that will increase your body's health and avoid foods that won't. UnDieting makes these decisions easy, as you'll quickly come to understand how simple it is to determine what is going to work for you and what will work against you.

✽ Say *Hey, how you been?* to the bit of yourself you keep just to yourself. Start to tap in to what you're really feeling and then allow yourself to tune into the attitudes that prompt you to eat. Pay attention to tension and emotions that may be affecting your eating patterns.

✽ Take note of when you feel naturally hungry. This is a tough one, as it is rare that we allow ourselves to feel hungry anymore. Just start to note the difference between a pure physical hunger and an emotional need or boredom.

✽ If your energy is low, consider whether you are feeling lethargic due to lack of movement and exercise versus a need for fuel from food. An inactive lifestyle is unhealthy for many reasons, but relating to food, we often look to food rather than physical exertion to pick up our energy.

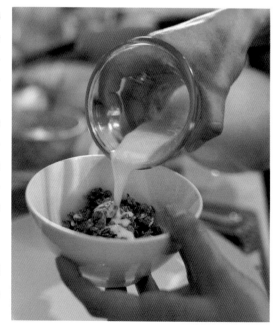

Let's not forget that the role of food is to fuel and nourish our sweet, beautiful selves. The first step in eating consciously: we have to slow this pony down.

YOUR CONSCIOUS EATING CHEAT SHEET ❀ Listen to your body ❀ Follow your intuition, not your cravings, to help you to make the right food choices ❀ Be discriminating when eating ❀ Eat when you feel natural hunger ❀ Be aware of your unconscious motivations when eating ❀ Eat to satisfy your physical needs, not your emotional ones ❀ Relax as much as possible before eating

Slow Down, Sally! This Isn't a Race

"Let's all just slow down." That's what my mom would tell us as kids (and as grown-ups, too), when it looked as though her hours in the kitchen were about to be inhaled in minutes. That she was a stay-at-home mom when my brother and I were growing up is about the only thing traditional about my family. We did always eat meals together, but our family tends to do things our own way.

When my niece, Mia Jean, was a toddler and needed a scheduled mealtime, my mom declared that we were now going to eat like Italians. To ensure we were at the table eating by 6:00 p.m. and to keep Mia from having a meltdown, what would normally be considered a complete meal — a salad, a couple veggie side dishes, a grain, and the main entrée — would now be enjoyed in five separate courses: a plate of salad, then a few pieces of broccoli, a spoonful or two of quinoa or brown rice, then a piece of fish and some sweet potato would round out the meal. Though perhaps a slightly (okay, completely) impractical and ridiculous option for slowing down the eating process, it was effective, and did invite us to eat a little less, linger longer at the table, and spend more time visiting.

With all the complaints about poor digestion, this should be the first thing we need to try: slowing down, chewing our food, breathing, resting, and digesting. This can't happen while stressing over our commute home, watching the latest horrors on the news, or eating while answering e-mails. Here are my three best reasons to slow down the food train.

❀ **Prevent Overstuffing Your Face.** It takes about twenty minutes for the message of satiety (that feeling that you have eaten enough), to reach your brain and to give you the old red light to stop eating. The more time you allow your brain to pick up that SOS signal from your belly, the better the chance of you stopping before you've gone too far. We have become used to defining the end of a meal as "feeling full." The more food we eat, the more work our digestive system has to do, and the more free radicals (see below) are produced as a natural byproduct of digestion and metabolism. The less we eat in volume (with more nutrition per bite) the better off we will be. Slowing down helps make that happen. The Okinawan people of Japan have a fantabulous practice called *hara hachi bu*, which means eating to 80 percent full. Say it a few times for fun. Then do it.

❁ **How Does That Taste? Pleasure At Its Best.** Ask yourself this question every time you take a bite. Take note of the texture of the food, the flavors in it, savor it, and love it. Focus on the food you are actually eating, rather than having your food be the activity to keep you entertained while focusing on something else.

❁ **Better Digestion.** If you are pooping out your last meal, and actually recognize what it was you had for that last meal, there's a problem. Digestion begins in the mouth – there are no teeth in the stomach. The digestion of carbohydrates commences in the mouth. Chewing releases saliva that is full to the brim with enzymes that start the digestion process. When you chew, a message is sent to your stomach, the main site of protein digestion, that it is game time, and it starts secreting the juicy goodness that will help digest your food when it lands in there. This creates an acid mix called *chyme* that will stimulate the pancreas and gall bladder to do their thing in the next stage of digestion.

Nice to Meet You, Grace! I don't mean a religious kind of grace, but if that suits you, go for it. This is about taking a moment before you eat to take a deep breath, give thanks to whomever or whatever you wish to thank – maybe the earth your salad was grown in, the farmer that tended to it, or the lover who prepared it – and the luxury of being able to choose the food you will be eating. That alone will bring you a little health bonus.

WHAT IS A FREE RADICAL ANYWAY? Free radicals are created from exposure to **pollution**, **stress**, lack of sleep, **toxins**, and **pharmaceuticals**, and are natural by-products of digestion. Remember when you were sitting by the campfire as a kid and a wee little **spark** jumped out of the fire and burned a mark into your fleece jacket? Well, that's similar to what **free radicals** do **inside our body**: they fly around, **causing trouble**. Where do **antioxidants** come in to the equation? Antioxidants are the **buckets of water** that quench out the **damaging effects** of free radicals. The more free radicals we have in circulation, the more antioxidants we need to fight the flames. Where do antioxidants come from? Eating **real food**, of course. **Berries**, spices, and **raw cocoa** are some of the most potent sources.

Tips for Slowing Down

* Sit down at a table (obviously) and focus on the food set before you.
* Take small bites and chew well.
* Put your utensils down between bites.
* No stuffing food into your mouth before you've swallowed the last mouthful.
* Check in once in a while as you're eating to see how you feel.
* Avoid eating in front of the TV, or while reading, walking, or driving.
* Eat at your own pace. It's not a race to see who finishes first.
* Eat with an attitude of gratitude, appreciating your food, where it came from, and the energy that went into getting it from the field onto your plate.

TOP SUPPLEMENTS TO IMRPOVE DIGESTION BY JOSH GITALIS

In addition to slowing down when we eat and avoiding overstuffing ourselves, there are natural remedies we can use to enhance our digestion. Try these out before resorting to any over-the-counter symptom suppressors.

* **Digestive Bitters:** Bitters have been used for thousands of years to stimulate and tone the digestive system. Typically in nature, plants that are poisonous have a bitter taste. As a survival mechanism our bodies ramp up all of our digestive processes to deal with the poison as effectively as possible to avoid getting sick. Herbalists observed this and used bitter herbs, such as dandelion root and gentian root, to achieve a similar effect. The best products combine a variety of bitter herbs.

* **Digestive Enzymes:** Enzymes help to break down the food that we eat. We have only one chance to break down food mechanically – by chewing. The rest is carried out by the enzymes that we secrete. A plant enzyme complex supplement is a great choice that works all along the digestive tract.

* **Probiotics:** Probiotic means "for life." These are the good bacteria that inhabit our digestive tract and one of their many jobs is to aid in the maintenance of healthy gut flora, vital for proper digestion.

* **Fiber:** Fiber comes in two forms: soluble and insoluble. They are both important for keeping us regular and keeping our insides clean.

* **L-glutamine:** Proteins are long chains of single amino acids. L-glutamine is an amino acid that is the primary fuel for all the cells that line our digestive tract. So it is extremely effective at healing an inflamed or damaged digestive tract like we see in people with Crohn's, colitis, or upper GI ulcers.

Josh Gitalis is an evidence-based clinical nutritionist who uses food and supplements therapeutically to heal the body and restore balance. He runs a private practice in Toronto.

ARE YOU GOING TO EAT ALL THAT?

All-you-can-eat buffets have always baffled me. Why on earth would I want to test my limits with an endless buffet? Quite frankly, the thought of indulging in as much food as my five-foot frame could keep down makes me want to yak. There is no good reason to ever eat or drink all you can. It never ends with a pretty picture and you know it too. We have all learned that lesson once or thrice.

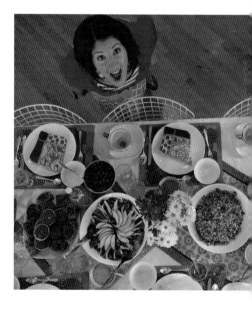

At the same time, I wish I could tell you that once you switch over to the whole and real foods of the UnDiet, you can eat to your overflowing belly and heart's content. Sadly, my sweet buffet devotee, this is not the case. Nuts are really healthy, but if you snack on nuts all day long, you will not wind up the picture of health. Raw honey is sweet and dandy; eat a whole jar and your teeth might jump out of your face. The adage *less is more* comes into effect when we're talking about food and setting a limit, a guideline if you will, on what is a reasonable amount to eat. We are eating more food, in volume and calorie count, than ever before. In 1964, the average North American consumed 2,947 calories per day. The average calorie consumption for 2015 is estimated to reach 3,440.[5] That's not a good thing. Without resorting to unhealthy practices such as weighing food or counting calories, we're going to take on a few of the following non-negotiables.

A Toast Plate for a Dinner Plate and a Soup Bowl for Salad

My mom, who is a potter, was once on a morning talk show presenting her beautiful ceramic work. As she was going through the different sized plates and platters she described one as a dinner plate and one as a toast plate. We've never let her forget it. But she was on to something. There's something to be said for eating meals on toast-size plates. We eat less.

We tend to fill our plate, no matter what the size. One of the easiest ways to cut back on portion size is to simply use a smaller plate and put less on it. The best tip to eat more goodness without feeling deprived is to use the biggest bowl (within reason) you can find and fill it with all the delicious greatness of fresh or lightly steamed veggies. Let this be your salad portion. Then grab that toast plate (or breakfast-size plate) and use that for your meal. Trust me on this one.

No More Sloppy Seconds

Fill your plate just once with all the delights you've made for dinner. Eat that portion mindfully, slowly, and with gratitude. Sip on some water; enjoy the conversation. Put your utensils down between bites. When that first serving is done, so are you. No second helpings. Can you dig it? And remember that your plate is now smaller, too. Double zinger. See, I told you there was no need to count calories. Just don't eat so much and we're all good.

Divvy up the Leftovers

It's tempting to put all your leftovers into one container; save space, and clean-up. It also allows you to dive into that massive container of leftovers and eat the whole thing with a fork, standing over your sink. Instead, portion out your leftovers so you have enough for two or three meals. Perhaps your leftovers can be topped up with salad or a whole grain, like quinoa or brown rice. Get creative. And just so you know, eating forkfuls of leftovers while you're putting them away, doesn't help anyone or anything. Just saying.

You also have to remember that these three pointers to reduce your overall intake are not punishable offenses when not followed strictly every single day for every single meal. They should be guidelines that you do your best to abide by, only letting them fall away when you absolutely have no choice.

Though I can't really think of a time when you would have no choice not to take seconds. Overindulging is always optional.

THREE MEALS FOR A REASON

Historians trace the whole three-meals-a-day thing back to the hoity-toity upper class and the evolving dining customs of British society. The North American version of the custom evolved with a few changes, where breakfast is grabbed on the go and dinner has become this massive weigh-you-down feast.

There is a common belief that we should be eating three meals a day and that breakfast is the most important meal. All true . . . sort of. Breakfast is an important meal, but so is dinner and so is lunch and so are your little snacks in between.

Please note, my hungry eaters, that *important* doesn't mean the same as *big*, or *heavy*, or *must be slaved over in the kitchen for hours*. Important means that the meal or snack you are about to consume has been given adequate thought and consideration. This attention has to go beyond what is the easiest, cheapest, and most convenient. We're not looking for a one-night stand here; we're looking for lifetime love. That little tripod of conditions tends to hold up most people's diet – and their subsequent health problems. It has replaced the considerations that should make up our food choices, which can be summarized in one word: *fuel*.

Yes, breakfast is the first drop of fuel in the tank for the day, after fasting overnight for eight to twelve hours, but everything we eat following breakfast tops up the tank. What we're aiming for with these three meals a day is to keep the tank filled and the engines running. The goal, of course, is that from a cellular level expanding out to our whole selves, our internal engine continues to purr like a sweet kitten being scratched behind the ears.

Ever experience that three o'clock sputter, crash, and clank where it feels like your muffler is dragging behind you? Or, put simply, have you ever felt so tired mid-afternoon that it takes all your effort not to shut your door, crawl under your desk, and sleep? That's what three meals a day are supposed to help prevent. The challenge, of course, is when our meals are easy, cheap, and convenient, and despite eating regularly, we aren't getting the real fuel our body needs from the food we're eating. We'll actually be missing the key components completely. The result of the easy and cheap thrills of processed convenience food is that we get energy spikes from all those refined ingredients, as opposed to the sustained long-burning energy we'd get from whole and healthy choices. The result: visits to the vending machine and coffee shop for that quick pick-up. We'll chat more about this in greater detail in Chapter 7. For the purposes of what we're talking about here, what you need to know is that you've got to center your meals and snacks on whole, real food. And eat regularly.

When we don't play by the three-meals-a-day (or five to six small meals) pattern, there are two categories many of us fall into: the mass consumer and the grazer.

The Mass Consumer

This usually occurs for people who don't wake up feeling hungry. Those of us who fall into this category tend to coast on nothing until lunchtime or even later, and then consume a big old giant meal. The problem is that our body is busy freaking out because it's not getting the fuel it needs first thing in the morning. The result: we go into hunter/gatherer famine mode and our metabolism slows down. Even if, calorie for calorie, we may not be eating that much, our body is hanging on to the calories for dear life, burning them as slowly as possible.

The Grazer

The opposite of the mass consumer is the grazer. This essentially means we munch on various things all the livelong day like cows out in pasture. The thing is, we're not cows. And if we graze for too long, we may just turn into one, in size at least.

We need our meals and snacks defined as such. Since we are now paying attention to our portion sizes and taking the time to eat our meals at a table intended for dining, we also need to acknowledge that there is a time when meal time is over. All those *just one more* and *just a little to tide me over* only feed those badass demons that, unfortunately, keep us from welcoming in the abundance of great health we are chasing.

The digestive system is a continuous tube that runs through us from top to bottom, or more specifically, from head to tail. An action in one part will directly affect the function in the next part down the tube. Ideally, we want the entire system to run its course from start to finish, meaning we eat, we digest, and our system has a chance to rest before we add more food into the mix. If you fall into the grazing category, this isn't happening.

Given the way the digestive system operates, for optimal function we need to take breaks between meals and step back from the trough. Whether you want to go with the three meals and two snacks or you prefer six small meals throughout the day, at some point, you just have to stop eating. Ideally, we want to aim to take at least a two- maybe three-hour break between meals. This gives our body a chance to run the full cycle of digestion with time to rest and replenish in order to get ready for the next round of goodness to come through.

POOPING AFTER MEALS If you've ever spent time with a **baby**, you have noticed that they tend to have a bowel movement after every **feeding** or meal. Their **systems** are primed and ready to go without having had any programming or emotional connections to their **digestive functions**. As we get **older**, we develop challenges, either having to **repress** the urge to use the bathroom or preferring not to use **public bathrooms** for doing number twos. Ideally, we want to have one meal in and one meal out. Most of us would be happy with **one good poop a day**. When things are moving well, typically you could expect the call of nature **within an hour** of completing your meal.

And while we're on the subject, late-night eating is just plain useless. The midnight snack of cookies and milk doesn't fit into the three- or six-meal plan. If you are hungry late at night, it probably means you're tired. You're mistaking the tired for hungry. Do yourself and your booty a favor and just go to sleep because that's what your bod is really signaling. And fasting for twelve hours a night, between dinner and breakfast, gives your digestive system a rest and lets your body use its energy for healing, repairing, and restoring so you can get up the next day and do it all over again with a skip in your step.

THE LOVE OF COMMUNAL DINING

I am pretty sure I am not alone in the fantasy of that dreamy Tuscan table set under an olive tree, with the vineyard off to the right and the organic garden to the left. Before us is a spread of fresh delights. Around the table is the most fantabulous gathering of friends and family as we eat, laugh, and chitchat.

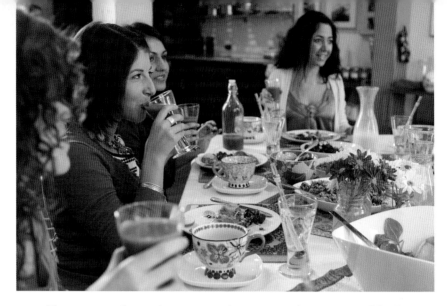

There is something inherent in us that craves gathering around food. Most cultures have rituals and ceremonies that involve food that bear significance to those who partake in the custom. Food and community are joined together through history, tradition, and necessity. I will forever question why my Eastern European Jewish roots have to include traditional foods such as *greben* (deep fried chicken skin) and *kugle* (a casserole of noodles, sour cream, and sugar).

If you ask me, a great big gathering of friends and food is the very best way to find the next best love of your life too, whether it is friends, lovers, or an introduction to new activities, books, movies, and ideas. There is a sharing that happens beyond what is on your plate; a lightness and joy that comes from celebration around a table where you are given little choice but to offer praise and thanks for the simplest things in life: love, health, and food. In this, family is formed.

Because many of us live worlds away from our families – whether it be physical location or lifestyle choices – family is often a feeling. We are born to relatives, but we have the ability to create our own families. So create the family of your dreams and do it simply, with fresh food. The communal dinner, or potluck, is a fantabulous way to employ all the gems of table manners. You are engaging in your food, engaging in each other, and are sitting down to dine at a table without the TV blaring.

A communal dining experience takes no more time to prep and prepare. All you have to do is make one dish and your peeps bring over the rest. Whether you meet weekly or monthly, this invites everyone to engage in conversation, create community, and nourish all aspects of life.

Do It at Work: Keeping healthy with a busy schedule can get tricky. To make it easier, bring others with you on the path of abundant health. Get a group of two to four peeps together at work, and assign each person one day of the week to prep and prepare snacks and lunches. If you get a group of five, that means you only have to think about lunch once a week. Awesometown easy, right?

UNDIET LIVING

UnDiet for Abundance Mantra
Slow down, Sally, this is meal time.

Make Love in the Kitchen
Eating is not an inconvenient chore or solution to boredom.

❋ No more multi-tasking while eating.

❋ Create a space at home and at work intended for dining only.

❋ Ditch the graze-a-thon between meals.

❋ Recognize your motivation for eating: hunger or emotion?

❋ Shut out the distractions (reading, TV, computer, walking, driving) when it is time for meals.

TRANSITIONAL TIPS AND TRICKS TO MAKE IT HAPPEN

❋ **Fill your plate just once. Not twice or thrice.**

Fill your plate with your meal and that's it, that's all. Pay attention to each bite, chew, chew more, swallow.

❋ **Put down your fork and slow down.**

Put down your cutlery between bites. This promotes proper chewing and slower eating. This one little change can reduce how much you eat and improve digestion.

❋ **Set the table with napkins and all.**

Dine at a table intended for dining for at least two meals a day. They will be enjoyed in the company of others, or alone, but without the distractions of a TV or computer.

❋ **Make time in your schedule.**

Set aside at least thirty undistracted minutes per day to eat your meals. That's just ten minutes per meal. I know you can do it.

❋ **Share a meal.**

At least twice per week, share a meal in a leisurely fashion with your friends and family, or get a group together at work and make meals a social and health supportive affair. Take the initiative and make sure it happens.

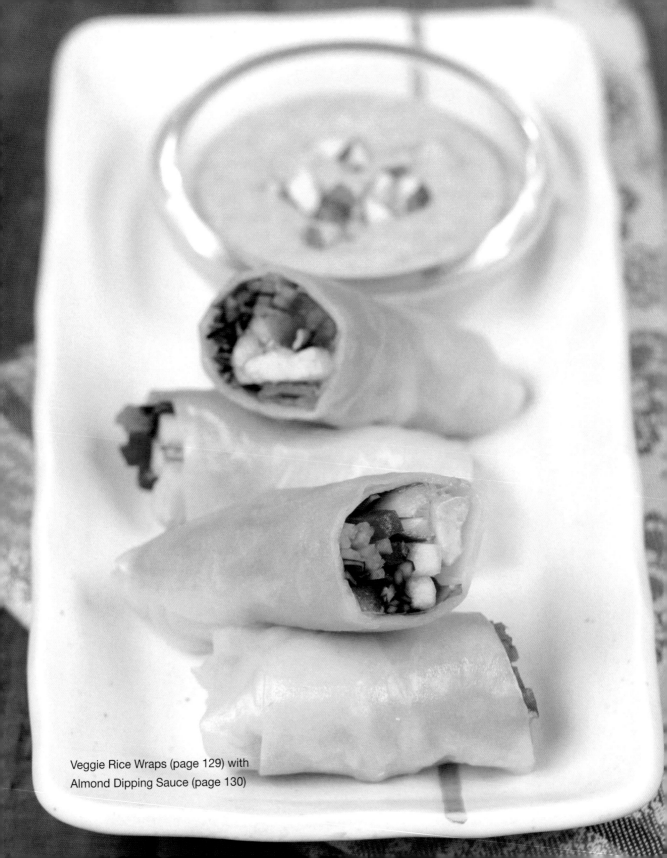

Veggie Rice Wraps (page 129) with
Almond Dipping Sauce (page 130)

Veggie Rice Wraps

Serves: 4 as a side, 2 as a meal

8	sheets rice paper	8
1	avocado, peeled and sliced lengthwise	1
1	carrot, grated	1
½	red bell pepper, sliced lengthwise	½
½	red apple, peeled and sliced into matchsticks	½
4 inches	cucumber, sliced into long strips	10 cm
1 cup	baby spinach	250 mL
¼ cup	cabbage, shredded	50 mL
2	organic eggs, whisked in a bowl, cooked as an omelet, then sliced into thin strips. (optional)	2
4	sprigs cilantro	4

DIRECTIONS

- Soak one piece of rice paper in warm water until soft. Carefully remove, allow excess water to drain, and lay out on flat surface.
- Arrange veggies in a row along center of rice paper. Add greens last. On your first few attempts, fewer veggies will be easier to roll.
- Leave about 1½ inches (4 cm) at both ends and carefully roll the wrap up, leaving long edges open. You'll take care of those with the second piece of rice paper.
- Soak and drain a second piece of rice paper, and lay out on flat surface. Place roll along center of second piece of rice paper, folding end edges in first and then roll in remaining sides.
- Serve with Almond Dipping Sauce (see page 130).

Pack It! If you make extras to take for lunch the next day, store in an airtight container with a slightly damp cloth or paper towel to help keep the rice wraps moist.

Almond Dipping Sauce

½ cup	almonds (or almond butter)	125 mL
¼ cup	water	50 mL
1 tbsp	lemon juice	15 mL
1 tbsp	maple syrup	15 mL
1 tbsp	tamari	15 mL
1	small garlic clove, minced	1
1 tsp	ginger root, grated	2 mL
	sea salt and cayenne to taste	

DIRECTIONS

❧ Put all ingredients in a food processor and process until smooth. You may need to scrape down the sides with a spatula and re-process.

Curried Caper Tahini Sauce

⅓ cup	tahini (sesame paste) or your favorite nut butter	75 mL
1 tbsp	maple syrup or raw honey	15 mL
2 tbsp	lemon juice	30 mL
2 tbsp	water	30 mL
2 tbsp	apple cider vinegar	30 mL
2 tsp	curry powder	10 mL
2 tbsp	small capers (packed in water)	30 mL
¼ cup	parsley, finely chopped	50 mL

DIRECTIONS

❧ Mix by hand or use a food processor to blend all ingredients together, adding water 1 tbsp (15 mL) at a time, until desired consistency is achieved.

❧ Serve with rice wraps or your fave burgers and sandwiches. Makes a great veggie dip too!

Thai Green Curry Paste

8	small green chilies, seeded and chopped	8
3	garlic cloves, minced	3
¼ cup	red onion, chopped	50 mL
2 cups	fresh cilantro leaves and stalks, coarsely chopped	500 mL
2 tbsp	ginger root, minced	30 mL
1 tsp	coriander seeds, ground	5 mL
1 tsp	turmeric	5 mL
1 tsp	ground cumin	5 mL
2 tsp	lime rind, grated	10 mL
½ tsp	sea salt	2 mL
1 tbsp	sesame oil	30 mL

DIRECTIONS

❧ Place all ingredients in a blender and process until smooth.

❧ Store in fridge for 1 week, or freeze in ice cube trays and then transfer to airtight container for 2 months.

Booyizzle White Bean Green Curry

Serves: 6

2 tbsp	cold-pressed extra-virgin coconut oil	30 mL
1	onion, finely chopped	1
3 tbsp	Thai Green Curry Paste (see page 130)	45 mL
2	garlic cloves, minced	2
1 cup	broccoli florets, cut into bite-sized pieces	250 mL
1 cup	cauliflower florets, cut into bite-sized pieces	250 mL
1 cup	carrots, sliced into thin coins	250 mL
⅔ cup	vegetable stock (see page 84) or water	150 mL
2	stalks lemongrass, bruised	2
15 oz	can organic white, kidney, or lima beans	425 g
1 cup	organic coconut milk	250 mL
1 cup	kale, woody stem removed, coarsely chopped	250 mL
1 cup	spinach, coarsely chopped	250 mL
½ cup	raw, unsalted cashews, coarsely chopped	125 mL
1	small bunch fresh cilantro	1
⅓ cup	fresh basil	75 mL
2 tbsp	lime juice	30 mL
½ tsp	sea salt or to taste	2 mL

DIRECTIONS

- In a medium saucepan, heat the coconut oil and sauté the onions for 5 minutes or until translucent. Add the curry paste and garlic and stir-fry for about 3 minutes.
- In a separate saucepan, steam broccoli, carrots, and cauliflower just until fork-tender, about 5 minutes.
- Add the stock or water and lemongrass to the onions, stir, then add the broccoli, cauliflower, carrots, and white beans. Simmer for 15 minutes until veggies are tender.
- Add the coconut milk, kale, spinach, and cashews and simmer another 5–8 minutes.
- Add the cilantro, basil, lime juice, and sea salt, and stir.
- Remove from heat and let sit for 10 minutes to meld flavors together, then remove lemongrass.
- Serve in large bowls, with noodles or brown rice, and garnish with fresh cilantro and a few chopped cashews.

Orange Zest–Infused Stew

Serves: 6

2 tbsp	extra virgin olive oil	30 mL
1	large red onion, diced	1
4	garlic cloves, minced	4
2 tbsp	ginger root, grated	30 mL
2 tsp	ground cumin	10 mL
2 tsp	ground coriander	10 mL
2 tsp	dried sage	10 mL
2 tsp	dried rosemary	10 mL
3	cinnamon sticks, 4 inches (2.5 cm) each	3
2 cups	sweet potato, cubed into ¾-inch (2-cm) pieces	500 mL
2 cups	butternut squash (or winter squash of choice), peeled and cubed into ¾-inch (2-cm) pieces	500 mL
1 cup	carrots, sliced into ¼-inch (5-mm) coins	250 mL
1 cup	parsnips, sliced into ¼-inch (5-mm) coins	250 mL
15 oz	can organic chickpeas, drained (or 2 cups cooked)	425 g
1	medium tomato, diced	1
⅓ cup	organic, sulphite-free apricots, chopped	75 mL
1 tbsp	organic orange zest	15 mL
2 cups	water	500 mL
2 tsp	arrowroot starch (optional)	10 mL
	sea salt and cayenne to taste	

DIRECTIONS

- Heat olive oil in a large pot over medium heat until warm. Add onion, garlic, ginger, cumin, coriander, sage, rosemary, and cinnamon sticks. Cook and stir for 5 minutes, or until onion is tender and translucent.

- Stir in vegetables, chickpeas, tomatoes, apricots, orange zest, and water. Bring mixture to a boil, reduce heat to medium-low, cover, and let simmer for about 30 minutes, stirring occasionally, until the veggies are tender.

- Remove lid and simmer for another 15 minutes. If it looks too watery, remove ½ cup (125 mL) of liquid and reserve in separate bowl. Whisk the arrowroot starch into this reserved liquid and then add it back to main saucepan.

- Once desired thickness is achieved, add sea salt and cayenne to taste.

- Remove the stew from heat, remove cinnamon sticks, and serve warm over quinoa, brown rice, or other whole grain.

> This stew freezes well. Once completely cool, transfer to ½- or 1-quart (½–1 liter) mason jars, leaving 3 inches (8 cm) of space at the top. Take the jar out in the morning to defrost and heat in a pan over the stove when you get home.

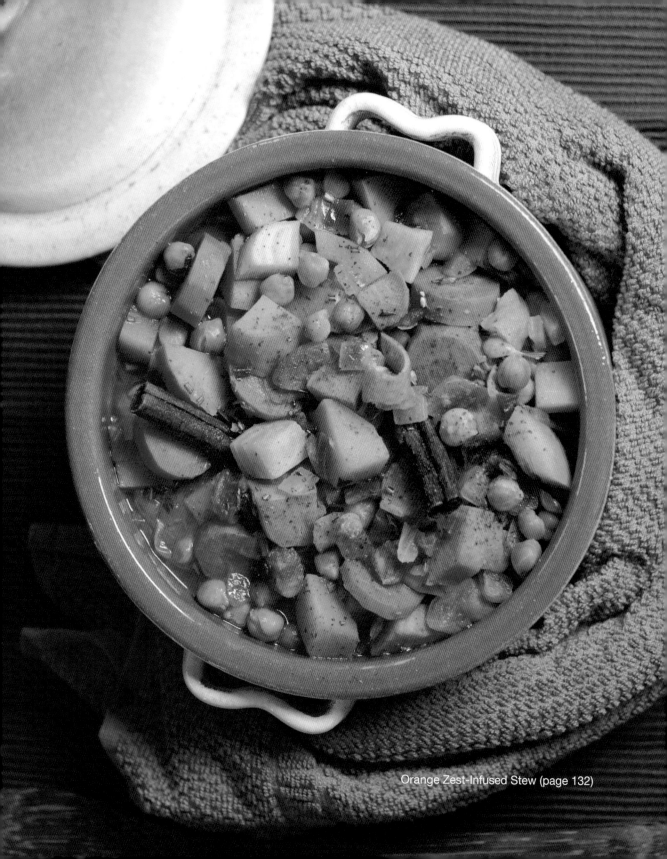

Orange Zest-Infused Stew (page 132)

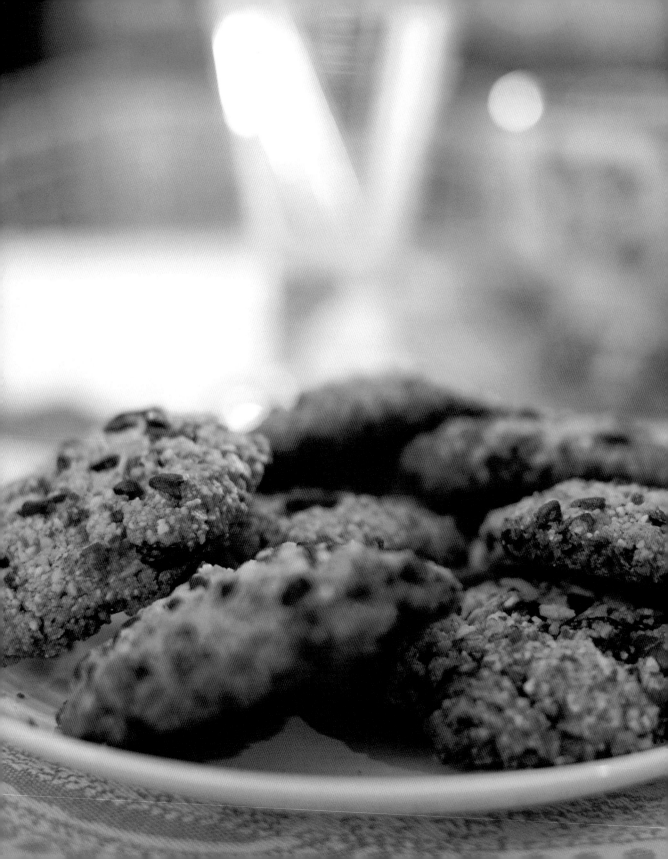

CHAPTER 7

Kicking the Cravings

It was June 2001 and I was in beautiful (and sweltering) Seville, Spain. This was long before the nauseatingly sweet smell of soda induced my overly sensitive gag reflex to activate, and long before I even knew what a nutritionist was. I had decided that I was going to put my vocabulary of approximately fifty Spanish words in to practice and spend the summer pretending to be one of the locals. In the midst of my solo gallivanting around Spain, my mom came out for a visit. We'd been touring all day in the midst of a heat wave. Following a delightful dinner of *tapas* (translation: small food . . . I think), we decided to hit the nightlife and grab a drink at a small bar. We were both so dehydrated and thirsty that, for some bizarre reason, we both ordered a Coke.

I was not raised on soda and I never drank it. I hated that fizzle-in-the-nose thing that would happen when you burped. Yet, in Seville and beyond any sane explanation, my mom and I sucked back our Cokes as if it were *ambrosia* (that's Spanish for ambrosia).

We went back to our room to sleep. Four hours later, we were both still wide awake, antsy-pantsy, reading the history sections of our guidebooks in the hopes that we'd bore ourselves to sleep. We were wired up like a double-D brassiere until the morning hours. Only later did I learn that one can of Coke can have as much as twelve teaspoons of sugar (think twelve sugar cubes or twelve times the amount that circulates in our blood stream) and loads of caffeine. Zingaling. No wonder we were up all night. The only thing worse than being up all night from caffeine is the barftastic furry feeling all that sugar leaves behind on the teeth.

TIME TO KICK IT ROOT DOWN

We're friends at this point, right? I've gained your trust. You like what I have to say, most of the time at least. You have been following the UnDiet for a few weeks now, and you're feeling good. Let's ruminate on all the love between us, how we're now old friends, comrades, and confidants, so that when I suggest that it may now be time for us to work together to kick some nasty habits, I know that we can battle the demons together and hug it out in the end. I am doing this for your own good, all out of love, I promise you.

One of the toughest things to do is to recognize our own bad habits, and even tougher is coming to recognize that something has to be done about them. It is usually our friends or family who will first bring them up to us, and in those moments, our immediate response might just be to disown those aforementioned friends and family, because, well, we didn't develop those bad habits intentionally. I don't know of anyone who wants to be hooked on a substance of any kind just to function. We tend to hang on to fulfilling our cravings, which develop into our habits, because we become afraid to give them up. On some level, we fear what life would be like without that thing, feeling, or experience. Somewhere, we have a story we like to tell ourselves that life is just better/happier/easier/_____ (fill in your blank here). Am I touching the soft spot yet, or are you off in mental defense mode with your fingers in your ears trying to silence me with your indignant humming?

You won't **achieve** your goal until you are **honest** about what's holding you back. Today is the day. Time to get those **cravings kicked** and those habits hitchhiking out of our lives.

The tricky part with any addictive habit, whether it is smoking, drinking coffee or alcohol, fulfilling that persistent chocolate craving, or sleeping in past your alarm, is that there is always an emotional connection as well as a physiological or chemical connection. This means that to successfully break any habits both the emotional and the physical elements of that habit must be addressed. It can be clear as a summer's day to see these habits in other people, likely those closest to us, but wowzers, you know that when you see these patterns in others, it is most often a sneaky-devil way for the universe to hold a mirror up to ourselves. Don't you dare go looking away.

The first step in breaking the bad habits and kicking those cravings is going to be recognizing what those things are. I will discuss some of the most common, coffee and sugar, but I will also invite you to throw your own pesky habits into the ring and battle it out.

Symptoms of Being Hooked on Bad Habits

There are many different bad habits and addictions, but similar symptoms tend to run the gamut. Since it can sometimes be tough to see that reflection of our not-so-shiny spots when we start digging down deep within, as you read through this section, pay special attention to what that mind of yours is spinning. Our mind has an amazing way of making us believe the web of tales as truth, when in reality, often it spins that web to simply allow us to continue believing that what we're doing is A-okay. Here are some symptoms to look out for:

✽ **Increased Tolerance:** Sometimes, the more we have of something, the more of it we tend to need to have the same desired response. This is where that one coffee in university turns into a half-dozen in the working world. The exception, of course, is the people who claim they just need one cup of coffee to get going and then they're fine. Who wants to rely on any substance to be "fine"?

✽ **Icky-Prickly Withdrawal:** Withdrawal is a word often used with slightly more dangerous substances than mocha lattes, cookies, and cakes, but if even the thought of removing any of those things from your diet promotes

"Every time you are tempted to react in the same old way, ask if you want to be a prisoner of the past or a pioneer of the future"
– Deepak Chopra

feelings of wanting to kick me in the taco, chances are that detoxing them from your life may be no walk in the park. Typically withdrawal symptoms are so uncomfortable because they produce the exact opposite feelings you are seeking by consuming that substance. For example, we drink coffee for alertness, and when we refrain we feel foggy. That fogginess is a withdrawal symptom.

❀ Getting the Goods Becomes Your Priority: This is when social, occupational, or recreational activities become more focused around your jonesing for the goodness. You make or alter plans in such a way that they enable you to get your fix. Your friend suggests a walk, and you suggest instead meeting to grab a cup of coffee.

❀ **You Make It Okay:** Sometimes knowing we shouldn't be doing something isn't enough. The sweet power of the brain enables us to rationalize that *just a little is fine,* or *after this row of cookies I'll stop,* or *this is the last time I'm buying that pint of ice cream,* or *tomorrow morning I'll get out of bed at seven and start my workout routine.* That *one more time* thought becomes your mantra, the recording you play every time, further enabling you to continue the habit. Lying isn't nice, especially to yourself.

THE OTHER ADDICTIVE WHITE POWDER: SUGAR

Sugar is more addictive than cocaine.[1] Don't believe me? There have been loads of studies done across this fair globe that prove its scary power. Most of us are introduced to sugar early in our lives, usually in the form of cake on our first birthday. From then on, it holds us in its spell, and may or may not play a leading role in our desire to read books with titles like UnDiet. Sugar, however, is far from harmless.

One study out of France, the land of wine and *la patisserie,* sought to prove that sugar is actually more addictive than cocaine.[2] Researchers on this study found that when rats were offered a choice between water sweetened with saccharin, an intensely sweet (and oh so neuro- and liver-toxic) artificial sweetener, and intravenous cocaine, 94 percent preferred the sweet taste of saccharin. Here you are thinking *of course they chose the insanely sweet substance over cocaine.* Here's the catch, though: the preference for saccharin could not directly be linked to its unnaturally intense sweetness. The researchers checked out the response with sucrose, a less intense, more natural sweetener, and had the same results. No matter if the substance was crazy sweet or subtly sweet, the rats went for it first.

When the rats were offered larger doses of cocaine, their preference for the sweetness of sugar water didn't waiver. Even rats addicted to cocaine switched to sweetened water when given the choice.

Another study from Princeton University, led by Professor Bart Hoebel, demonstrates the effects of sugar bingeing and deprivation in rats.[3] In Hoebel's study, rats that were denied sugar for a prolonged period after learning to binge on it would work harder to get it when it was reintroduced to them. His team found that the rats consumed more sugar than they ever had before, suggesting this was craving and relapse behavior. When their supply had been cut off and then reintroduced, their motivation for sugar had only increased. Yikes! That doesn't bode well with our *just a taste won't hurt* rationalizing strategy.

Interestingly, in this same study, it was found that with their supply of sweet white sugar cut off, the rats drank more booze, demonstrating that the bingeing habit with the sugar may have actually altered the way their brains were working. The researchers noted that these affected brain functions served as "gateways" to other paths of destructive bingeing behavior. Hoebel and his posse also found that the brain chemical that makes us feel easy, breezy, calm, and squeezey, called dopamine, was released in a region of the brain known as the *nucleus accumbens* when the rats drank the sugar solution. This chemical release is believed to trigger motivation and, eventually, with repetition, addiction. This explains why a sugar addiction can have such an emotional response. We feel good when we have it, and cranky when we need it.

This is probably freaking you out right now, but that's okay. We're moving through it together and we're gonna kick the habit together, too.

THE BLOOD SUGAR WATERFALL
INTO THE RIVER OF ADRENALINE

I know comparing sugar to narcotics is rather extreme for our fun-loving walk through abundant living. Sometimes though, we have to know some facts to help us pull our socks up and get us walking in the right direction.

The thing is, it's not just white sugar that hooks us. All refined and processed food has the ability to make us powerless slaves to our cravings and I am going to explain precisely why, despite our best intentions, we don't always have the best follow through.

❀ **Blood Sugar Level:** Also known as blood glucose level, our blood sugar level is a measure of how much circulating glucose we have in our blood. An imbalance can result in a hyper- or hypoglycemic state — both of which can result in severe symptoms that can lead to death.

❀ **Insulin:** This is a hormone produced in the pancreas that is vital for metabolizing fat and carbs. Insulin helps the cells of the liver muscles and fat tissue take glucose from the blood and convert it into stored energy called glycogen. Too much insulin will block the body's use of glycogen for energy, which in turn will result in more glucose being converted into junk in the trunk rather than glycogen.

❀ **Adrenaline:** Also known as epinephrine, adrenaline is a hormone and neurotransmitter that, in addition to helping keep our blood pumping and our lungs breathing, is critical in short term acute stress responses in the sympathetic nervous system.

❀ **Cortisol:** Produced in the adrenal glands, cortisol is a hormone that plays a role in responding to stress and helping to restore balance. Prolonged cortisol secretion (often due to poor diet and/or chronic stress) can have severe long-term physiological implications, including increased inflammation, weight gain, and reduced immune response.

Most of us wake up in the morning with our blood sugar slightly low.

This, of course, is totally normal, because we've been fasting all night. We have a bite to eat in the morning, perhaps some toast, or a muffin, some orange juice, and maybe a cup of coffee to get us going. Our blood sugar level spikes as a result.

When we have more sugar in our blood stream than we can actually get into the cells and convert to energy, our insulin levels spike. Insulin is the hormone secreted by the pancreas that acts as the sugar shuttle. If that sugar stays in our blood stream too long, we get hyperglycemic, which can lead to shock and become deadly. High insulin levels, however, put our body in a sluggish, fat-storing metabolic mode. Ongoing abuse of insulin is linked to increased risk of type 2 diabetes, heart disease, obesity, and cancer.

With high amounts of insulin circulating, working to get that sugar out of our blood, our blood sugar levels often experience rather dramatic drops. This is the sugar crash that leads us to the river of adrenaline. Remember: what goes up must come down. This means that around eleven in the morning, we go on the hunt. Maybe we grab another coffee, or start counting down the seconds until lunch.

Meanwhile, this sugar crash has us now operating in a bit of a stressed state, the old "fight or flight" you may recall from earlier. With our blood sugar dropped, our adrenaline kicks in, and suddenly we feel hyper alert, perhaps impatient, irritable, and anxious, with an increased heart rate. We have our lunch of pasta, pizza, a sandwich, or maybe the white-rice sushi from that great place down the street. Perhaps it's followed by a sweet treat, and by three in the afternoon we are feeling more tired than ever in our life. We have crashed again, and we're seeking the vending machine. Sugar, of course, becomes the quick fix to pick our energy back up, and there we are, back in that cycle. Later in the evening, we experience a third (fourth? Fifth?) wind and are suddenly buzzing around until late night, our head spinning.

That 4:00 a.m. wake-up, my dear friend, is adrenaline knocking on the door of your unconscious mind telling you it is ready to play. You have been riding this adrenaline roller coaster for too long and that is the cycle we want to break. Elevated adrenaline levels don't just have short-term effects. Adrenaline is the stress hormone that is meant to kick in and help us get through periods of short-term acute stress. The challenge, as I explained in Chapter 6, is that we are using this gem of a hormone all too often and, oh man, is it a powerfully addictive substance. It's the hormone people go bungee jumping and skydiving for. It's a rush. Long-term abuse, however, will cause long-running elevated levels of cortisol. Cortisol is our other stress hormone, intended to helps us cope with long-term chronic stress: everything from injury recovery to caring for a loved one. Long-term elevated levels, however, will also lead to long-term deteriorating health problems such as chronic inflammation, hormone imbalance, and weight gain – but I'll get to that.

A normal **blood sugar** level is slightly less than one teaspoon of sugar dissolved in all of our body's blood. As Dr. Michael Eades explains, an order of medium fries can contain up to 47 grams of refined carbohydrate, equivalent to almost ten teaspoons of sugar.[4] Eating the fries increases our blood sugar to **ten times more** than a **normal blood sugar** level. One quarter of a teaspoon is all the difference between normal blood sugar and that of a diabetic. Ten full teaspoons would be **forty times** that amount. The increased insulin required to get the sugar out of the blood affects our **hormonal system,** which leads to a slower metabolic rate and an increase in belly fat.

Disease, I will remind you, is not something we catch. It is something that we build over time: piece by piece, habit by habit. We don't catch type 2 diabetes or heart disease. We don't catch being fat or having a hormonal imbalance. You can't catch low thyroid function, impaired mental processing abilities, or even cancer. We build these things over time, through various lifestyle habits. Obviously we may have an inherent weakness or genetic predisposition to certain conditions, but they are not life sentences and they are also not inevitable.

Your shoes will wear out much faster if you wear them every single day than if you rotate between a few pairs, right? If we abuse our body, we will wear it out faster. Chronically riding the insulin, adrenaline, and cortisol waves will take its toll with long-term and lasting chronic conditions.

LONG-TERM EFFECTS OF ABUSING OUR STRESS HORMONES

* **Weight Gain:** Belly fat, or "the spare tire," is associated with hormonal imbalances resulting from elevated insulin, cortisol, and adrenaline levels.

* **Fatigued Adrenal Gland Function:** The adrenal glands, which sit just above our kidneys, help us cope with stress. When we abuse them and run them out of juice, we experience anxiety, depression, PMS, headaches, chronic fatigue, emotional swings, and other cranky-pants fun.

* **Impaired Mental Health:** Long-term abuse of stress hormones will impair thought, perception, memory, and concentration. Essentially, you stop seeing and processing life as it is.

* **Suppressed Thyroid Function:** Resulting from imbalanced hormones, we get impaired thyroid function. This can result in muscle stiffness, chronic exhaustion, morning nausea, hair loss, insomnia, weight gain, diminished sex drive, recurrent infections, depression, multiple food allergies/sensitivities, cystic breasts, and menstrual irregularities. Hey, you sexy thing!

* **Insulin Resistance/Type 2 Diabetes:** When we abuse our cells by throwing heaps of insulin at them, there will come a point where they say no (often referred to as insulin resistance), or need more than we can produce (what we'd call insulin dependence). The overall result is an inability to regulate blood sugar levels, a potentially deadly state.

* **High Blood Pressure:** Stress is not good for the heart, physically or emotionally. With a reduced ability to process it, we feel stress on a physical level more acutely, leading to high blood pressure, which in turn is commonly associated with blood clots, heart attacks, and strokes.

* **Lowered Immune Response:** There is nothing worse for our overall health than stress. Again, the abuse of stress hormones impairs the function and efficiency of the immune system. This means that anything, from

recovery from the common cold, post-surgery recuperation, to dealing with autoimmune conditions is more severe, takes longer, and is tougher on our bodies.

❀ **Increase in Inflammatory Conditions:** Cortisol is the body's in-house anti-inflammatory. Too much use and abuse and there isn't enough to do its job, which can result in rheumatoid arthritis, colitis, autoimmune conditions, skin conditions, allergies, and asthma, as well as a lower pain threshold over time.

FOODS THAT SPIKE BLOOD SUGAR

Refined and processed carbohydrate foods with a side helping of coffee and alcohol are the foods that are going to use and abuse your blood sugar levels, leading to the aforementioned cascade of health disasters. Before you hop on the protein-only bandwagon and start consuming copious amounts of meat, Gabriel Cousens, a leader in whole-food, plant-based, and raw diets for reversing diabetes, explains that a quarter pound of meat has the same insulin load as a quarter-pound of sugar.[5] Both release dopamine, creating that addiction. The trick then is not to drop all carbs, go fad diet

The Digestion Breakdown:
You Eat a Honey-Glazed, Jelly-Stuffed Donut

❀ No digestion is needed by the body (refined flour is essentially like pure sugar or glucose).

❀ Blood sugar levels surge into bloodstream and peak.

❀ Pancreas secretes insulin to help get sugar into cells.

❀ Blood sugar level drops dramatically.

❀ Adrenal glands kick in and secrete adrenaline to pick level back up, and coritsol is secreted. This results is a complete stress response: our heart races, our mood fluctuates, and our digestion grinds to a halt.

❀ Adrenaline levels peak and then crash.

❀ You crave more sugar and reach for another donut.

on me and just eat meat. We're going to do this intelligently by getting rid of the refined carbohydrate foods, which include: fruit juice, muffins, cookies, cake, donuts, white bread (bagels, baguettes, pitas), pasta, white rice, all-purpose flour, and rice cakes, to name a few. Additionally, coffee and booze are going to have to go, due to their stimulating effects on our stress levels and insulin output.

Most of the foods listed above (aside from coffee) are what we would call "simple carbohydrates," short little chains of sugars that require minimal digestion for the sugar to rush the blood stream. Alternately, whole foods like beans, legumes, whole grains, nuts and seeds, and leafy green vegetables, though they have carbohydrates in them, are "complex carbohydrates," which means the sugars come in longer chains. With complex carbohydrates, the body needs to break up more of the bonds in these chains to get the sugar. The result is that the sugar is absorbed more slowly, taken up by the cells as the sugar enters the blood stream, less insulin is required by the body to process that sugar, and our stress hormones, adrenaline and cortisol, aren't called into action.

THE CAFFEINE DITCH

The caffeine ditch is something we can fall into and have a tough time climbing out of. Don't worry; I've got my rope ladder at the ready for you.

My clients often ask me, *Is coffee really that bad for me?* The answer may surprise you. No. It's not that bad for you. There is, of course, a catch. The catch is that coffee is great, delicious, and a treat, when consumed once in a while, as an occasional indulgence. If, however, you are more closely related to zombie than human before you slurp back your morning brew, then my answer is, *Yes, coffee really is that bad for you.*

Our collective goal, yours and mine, with this whole vibrantly healthy UnDiet thing we've got going on here, is that we want to do our best to not have to rely on any substance except maybe real food, water, sunshine, and fresh air to function. Just as it is not ideal to be chained to a medication, we also wouldn't want to be chained to a voluntary substance such as coffee or sugar. Moderate amounts of caffeine, in a relaxed setting, when in fine and dandy health, is no problem. This, however, is not how most of us are drinking it, and many of us, if under any kind of stress, become even more sensitive to it.

So how are we going to get out of the caffeine ditch? I am sad to say that there is no real easy way to detox from caffeine. It's hard. It's likely gonna suck, but the freedom you will experience when you are able to wake up and float out of bed in the morning and be calm and clear headed all the live-long day will be well worth the challenge. Need convincing?

Caffeine causes a cascade of processes in our body to run amok. Let's look at some of them.

Caffeine and Hormones

Caffeine has a half-life of four to six hours, which means it is kicking around in our body, predominantly our nervous system, for a long time. It affects the functioning of a whole cocktail of hormones, including:

✢ **Adenosine:** This hormone helps calm the body. Caffeine inhibits its absorption. This is, in part, why we feel alert in the short term, but have sleep problems later on.

✢ **Adrenaline:** The hormone that fuels our workforce! Caffeine injects adrenaline into our system, offering a temporary boost. But what goes up must come down, leaving us feeling fatigued and depressed. What do we do then? Grab a second cup. Sipping up more caffeine to counteract these effects leaves us feeling agitated and edgy.

✢ **Cortisol:** The "stress hormone" that is supposed to help us cope with long-term chronic stress gets played out with caffeine consumption. Elevated cortisol is associated with weight gain and moodiness, and over the long run it has been associated with heart disease, diabetes, and cancer. Boo!

✢ **Dopamine:** Caffeine increases this feel-good hormone's levels in the body (as does sugar), acting in a way similar to amphetamines. Yikers! Unfortunately, once it wears off, we are left feeling rather low, which contributes to that physical dependence.

Caffeine and Sleep

We know caffeine keeps us awake, but that wakefulness doesn't always fade away that quickly. Once our stress hormones are activated, they tend to have their way with us. The effects of caffeine on our stress hormones can impair the mighty restorative deep-sleep cycles. This in turn affects the strength of our immune system, as well as levels of alertness the next day, and there we are, back in the caffeine dependence cycle.

Caffeine and Stress

Caffeine increases our stress levels, from perceived stress in our external world to the stress response we have on the inside. Stress and caffeine can elevate cortisol levels, which can lead to other negative health effects, including accelerated aging and anxiety. Increased levels of cortisol lead to crazy cravings for caffeine, fat, and carbohydrates, and so the cycle continues.

THE SLIPPERY COFFEE SLOPE

Does this mean you have to give up your occasional weekend latte or what have you? No, not yet at least. You just don't want to have to depend on it. This does mean, however, that if this is one of the cravings you are kicking, then together we say "later, latte," and get over the addiction before we can indulge in the occasional double-espresso, grande, extra-hot, vanilla-bean, milk-free, backwards-flip, upside-down, mocha, frappe, chilled, latte.

READY TO KICK THE BAD HABIT AND ELIMINATE THE CRAVINGS?

First we're going to address the general bad habit, crave-kicking needs. These are guidelines to help kick any craving or bad habit that is not serving our highest and bestest self. This includes sugar and coffee, but can also include hitting the snooze button eighty-five gazillion times, skipping your workout, late-night snacking, forgetting to floss your teeth, and everything in between. Instead of taking on all your habits at once, start with just one habit you want to kick, tackle that one, and move on to the next.

We're looking for abundance and goodness here, not torture-chamber-style cranky-pants misery.

Step 1: Define and Commit

This might be the toughest step of all. If you're anything like me and have a history that involves loads of different jobs and loads of different people you dated who you thought you might marry one week and who you left in the dust the next, well, defining what you want and committing to it may be the toughest step. See, you can't make changes for anyone else. You have to do it first and foremost for your own sweet, lovely, and oh-so-deserving self. The track record shows that people who acknowledge, on their own terms, that they need to move and shake things up a little in their life are far more likely to win the gold medal of empowerment by actually doing it, compared to the peeps who attempt something because they've been nagged into it. Change is hard, but taking active baby steps will move you closer to kicking the nasty habit to the ground. It will just require commitment and dedication.

❀ **Task: Define very specific behavior goals, and tailor your activities and attitude to make it work.** For example, if you're trying to cut out chocolate cake, and every Saturday night you eat at the same restaurant that makes the most amazing chocolate cake, then perhaps you should try dining somewhere else. If you want to start waking up at 7:00 a.m., then make efforts to go to bed before 11:00 p.m.

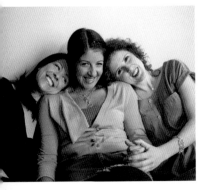

Step 2: Lean On Me (or Someone Else You Know and Love)

You can't always fix things all by your lonesome. When it comes to kicking habits (or perhaps we need to start looking at it as "creating new ones"), get a posse together. It can be a real-life BFF right-next-door kind of posse, or you can create a virtual one with peeps online from across the land. (Twitter can be great for finding people with the same goals as you — just search #UnDiet and you'll see what I mean.) The bottom line here is don't do it alone. Get yourself a little help. The help could be in the form of having someone or a group of people work to achieve the same goal together, a more formal support group, or even a specific coach or counselor. This may also mean, however, changing up the company that you keep. Quitting bad habits is no easy feat, and it is not made easier by spending time during your witching hour with people who are still enjoying whatever you may be trying to give up or change.

✽ **Task: Get that support posse together.** Whether they're real people you can meet through your gym or yoga studio, work, family, or greater community, or people you connect with online, or a health coach, counselor, or therapist — just choose wisely and have them cheerleading your success and also positively reinforcing your efforts in the event that you have setbacks. Note that when it comes to setbacks, you want your posse to throw tough love your way, tell you what you need to hear, and steer you back on the rails.

Step 3: Make a Timeline

When it comes to making major shifts in your lifestyle, there is no need to make it to home base on your first time up to bat. Like making out with your first boyfriend, you want to spend a little time at each base, taking it from first to second and enjoying each experience and adventure, no matter how anxious you may be about how far you go. The key to success in breaking the bad habits is to establish clear and realistic sub-goals and timelines. If kicking bad habits was easy peasy, we wouldn't have them in the first place. Chart your progress in a diary or calendar that outlines a realistic amount of time to eliminate the bad habit. If you are guzzling down a half-dozen mugs of caffeine each day, cutting it out 100 percent straight away is going to hurt. Cut down two cups a day one week, the next week you take it down by one more, and so on.

✽ **Task: Pick your goal date of being free of that habit, and work your way backwards in your timeline.** Choose specific milestones you want to reach by a certain time and aim for them. If you miss one, that doesn't mean you failed and get to give up. The F-word is not an option. A good goal to start with is to make it to twenty-one days free and clear of the habit, and at ninety days you best be having a major celebration.

Step 4: Remove and Replace

The most effective way to begin any lifestyle transition is to add something in for everything you take away. Let's pretend your bad habit is watching TV at night. If your goal was to cut out one hour of TV every night, you wouldn't just sit on the sofa with the TV off, staring at the blank screen. Fill that time with other fun-loving, vibrant-living activities, such as sleep or knitting me some pink mittens. The point being, when you remove one habit from your life, it's a good idea to have another great one ready and waiting to take its place. Adding a competing desirable behavior to compensate for the elimination of the bad one helps to overcome any void that may be initially felt. We need something to take the place of a habit to help us keep our eye on the goal.

❋ **Task: Determine what good things or activities are going to take over for the bad.** Replace the bad habits with good ones and do so before new bad habits find their way in to the mix.

Step 5: Get Up When You Fall Down

It's okay to have an oopsy-daisy once in a while; just don't make the slip-ups a regular occurrence. Know that you can't be perfecto all the time, but also know that eating one piece of chocolate cake when you promised yourself you wouldn't doesn't mean that you can go and eat the entire cake. One cup of coffee doesn't mean you get to go back to mainlining the caffeine. You also can't stress about the little upsets. That stress will likely hold your hand and walk you back down the path you've been walking forward on.

❋ **Task: Plan ahead.** If you know that you will find yourself somewhere that has a big flashing "temptation ahead" sign, then plan your defenses in advance. Remember that you've come this far, you've made this commitment, and you are sticking with it. Defensive strategies, along with your iron will, can help keep the backslides to a minimum.

Step 6: Reward Yourself!

Yay, you! Whenever you reach your milestones, or have a great moment, a great day, or a great week, make it count. That little reward center of the brain loves a good old massage and cuddle. Keep in mind that a great day does not equal a cheat. Not eating sugar for a whole week doesn't mean you get a whole day to eat as much as you can stuff in your face. You'll never get the old chocolate chip off your shoulder if you keep putting it back there every week. The reward should be in line with your goals. Maybe it's going for a massage, getting a mani-pedi, buying a new book, or a new ball of yarn for that pink scarf you're knitting for me as a thank-you gift. Just keep on acknowledging your accomplishments and rewarding yourself as you go.

❋ **Task: Use your reward as your motivation.** Plan out some rewards along the way to give you that extra little kick in the bottom to keep plugging away at your bad-habit-kicking goals.

CURB THOSE CRAVINGS

Now that you're ready to rock and roll away those bad habits, I am here, at your service, to offer some key tips to assist in breaking bad habits as they relate to the goodness we eat. Often, despite our very best of the best intentions, we become derailed when the cravings hit. It's hard. Sugar is just one of our most common addictions, but there are loads more. Eating in front of the TV or in the car, grabbing the wrong snacks, or making poor meal choices in a moment of desperation are also common goal bombers. This is where Steps 4 and 5 come in to play. You need to have strategies in place and plan ahead.

Tips for Curbing Those Cravings

❋ **Eat Regularly:** Eat three meals and two snacks or five to six small meals a day. This goes back to our earlier convo about keeping that blood sugar balanced. When the blood sugar takes a nose dive, we may get a little crazed, and next thing we know we're covered in crystallized sugar from those darn addictive sour jelly candies. The challenge is that the prickly, uncomfortable, cranky feelings of blood sugar crashes are immediately relieved by the consumption of sugar. The more refined, the better, so sticking to your goals feels almost impossible. Have no fear. Since we're kicking it with real food now, and committing to eating regularly, we're smooth sailing.

❋ **Protein, Fat, and Fiber With Every Meal and Snack:** Healthy sources of each will help keep your blood sugar stable. If you're having an apple, throw some almond butter on top. If you're making a smoothie, drop some hemp seeds, chia seeds, or your fave non-soy, non-dairy protein powder into the blender. You don't need a lot of the protein, fat, and fiber, but you do need a good quality source.

❃ **Choose Real, Whole Foods:** I doubt you need another reminder as to why you have to eat the goods as straight from the earth as possible with minimal chemical intervention. Here's your reminder: the closer a food is to its original form, the less processed sugar it will contain, and the more nutrients that will still be intact. It's those nutrients our bods really want, but we somehow mistake the craving for straight up processed salt or sugar. Food in its natural form generally helps to keep the blood sugar and mood stable and sweep those cravings under the bamboo rug.

❃ **Supplements:** Supplements are not meant to replace a good diet. They are intended to *supplement* proper eating by adding a little extra dose of nutrition when we need it. Detoxing from bad habits might mean we need a little extra love and care from some high-concentration nutritional supplements. A good-quality multivitamin (one you buy at a health food store, not a pharmacy brand full of corn and sucralose), along with a multi-mineral supplement, vitamin D, and a good dose of omega-3 essential fatty acids will help to support your nervous system and give your mood a sweet little boost. You want to make sure you are topping up those nutrients, as nutrient deficiencies can actually make cravings worse. If you are putting together a little supplement plan, you're likely best off chatting with your fave natural health care practitioner.

One and the Same Poison: Be careful when reading package labels – high fructose corn syrup often falls under the name "glucose/fructose." Don't be fooled.

❃ **Undercover Sugar:** Often foods we think of as whole and healthy are really refined carbohydrates, or simple sugars, in disguise. These are things such as orange juice and brown bread. Read the ingredient lists. Whole-wheat flour is not the same as whole-grain flour; glucose/fructose is not the same as a whole orange. You see what I'm getting at? Chances are good that as soon as the food has gone through some kind of processing, those sugars have been broken down and will cause blood sugar imbalance.

❀ **Add Spice to Your Life:** You know there is more that we can use to season our food than just pepper and salt, right? Coriander, cinnamon, nutmeg, cloves, and cardamom will naturally sweeten your foods and reduce cravings. Cinnamon is one of the über best at actually helping to balance blood sugar. Add cinnamon to your porridge, cumin to your dips, cloves to your baked goods, and brew them up together for a wicked tea.

❀ **Shake Your Groove Thang:** Walk, run, dance, sun salute (um . . . that means yoga), jump on the bed, chase your lover around the house naked. Do whatever you love most and do it. Just move. Moving around helps release tension and stress. Moving, even if just for five or ten minutes, can also change how we feel enough to make the craving a thing of the past.

❀ **Catch Your Zzzzs:** When we're pooper shnickled and can't seem to get our bootay in gear, processed sweets tend to find their way into our hands. Getting enough sleep will not only help fuel your energy levels, but will also help to provide that little bit of force to keep your will power intact. When we're tired, it's much harder to stave off the craving monster. From now on, let it be my voice. And what is my voice saying? *Toughen up! I know you can. You are better than this.* And then I make a one-person human pyramid in your honor. Fun! Now get your rest so you have the energy to human pyramid with me.

❀ **Be Willing to Get Right Down to the Emotion:** This might be the toughest bit of all, but being open to looking into the emotional goo can help us to extinguish that emotional need we often experience that makes us want to get a hug and kiss from a pint of ice cream. Get it on (not like that) with your support posse, journal it, draw some pictures, or compose a song on the old guitar. Knowing where to start in order to release the goo can be sticky; try a few strategies until you find what works for you.

A REMINDER OF SOME OTHER THINGS WE COVERED

Don't even think about forgetting the stuff we discussed together in earlier chapters. At times like these it is most important that you keep following them.

❧ **Keep Your Cupboards Clean of the Temptation:** If you don't have it in your home or office, you're less likely to eat it.

❧ **Never Substitute with Artificial Sweetener:** Ever. Is that clear?

❧ **Read the Ingredients, Not the Health Claims:** Those health claims are created by very smart men and women, likely while sipping on caffeinated drinks and eating donuts. Don't fall prey to their marketing wizardry.

❧ **Become Familiar with Sugar Terminology:** No matter what the kids are calling it these days — corn syrup, corn sugar, high-fructose corn syrup, sucrose, dextrose, glucose, fructose, beet sugar, raw sugar, cane sugar, molasses, turbinado sugar, or brown sugar — it's still all sugar.

SWEET ALTERNATIVES

There are sweeteners out there that are healthier, containing minerals still intact and possessing certain healing properties as well. This doesn't mean we should go crazy and use them on anything and everything, but during those times we want a treat, have these on hand so you can bake yourself something special. Most of these are easily found at your local health food store.

❧ **Raw Honey:** Unpasteurized (raw) honey contains many phytonutrients, antimicrobial, antiviral, and antioxidant properties. Raw honey also contains probiotics, the friendly bacteria that is beneficial for our gut and immune system. Substances in raw honey have been shown to prevent cancer and the development of tumors. Don't be fooled by the always liquid pasteurized honey at the grocery store that comes in a plastic beehive-shaped container. The processing and heating of honey destroys its magical powers.

❧ **Palm Sugar:** This is the crystallized nectar of the coconut palm flowers (originating from the coconut palm tree). Palm sugar is low on the glycemic index so it won't have our blood sugar soaring. It boasts high levels of potassium, magnesium, iron, zinc, vitamin C, and many B vitamins.

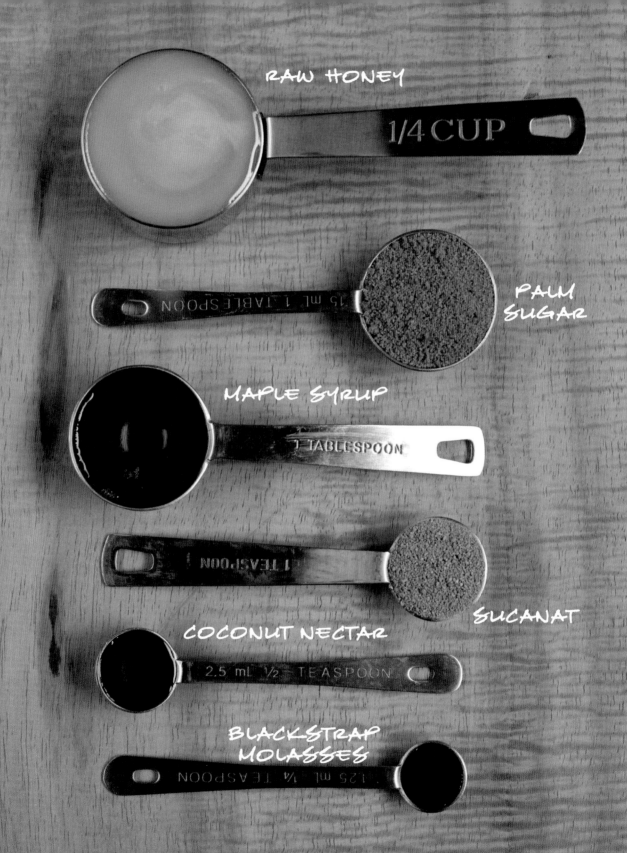

RAW HONEY

PALM SUGAR

MAPLE SYRUP

1/4 CUP

15 mL 1 TABLESPOON

1 TABLESPOON

1 TEASPOON

SUCANAT

COCONUT NECTAR

2.5 mL ½ TEASPOON

BLACKSTRAP MOLASSES

1.25 mL ¼ TEASPOON

❀ **Maple Syrup:** Made from the sap of the maple tree, it is high in manganese and zinc: two minerals important for proper immune function. Among many functions, zinc helps keep our men's prostates healthy and manganese us fertile as it lends a helping hand in the production of sex hormones.

❀ **Sucanat:** Sucanat is sugar-cane juice that is clarified, filtered, and evaporated. The syrup then crystallizes. This still retains the vitamins and minerals present in the sugar cane itself. It is sweeter than sugar: therefore we can use less of it.

❀ **Coconut Nectar:** This is a great alternative to the more common agave. It scores very low on the glycemic index, which means it will have minimal impact on your blood sugar levels, and it contains seventeen amino acids. Rich in B vitamins and vitamin C, it's also chock full of enzymes. I love using coconut nectar in smoothies and drizzled over ice cream or apples as a replacement to caramel sauce.

❀ **Blackstrap Molasses:** This thick black syrup is actually the by-product from the process of refining sugar cane into table sugar. What is left is a plethora of nutrients. Molasses is a super source of iron and actually provides more iron for fewer calories in comparison to red meat. It is also a great source of calcium to keep our bones healthy, regulate enzyme activity, and aid in nerve function.

❀ **Stevia:** This sweetener comes from the stevia plant and is calorie-free. It has phytonutrients, minerals, vitamins, and volatile oils. It is also believed to have antibacterial and antimicrobial properties. As it is not an actual sugar source, it has no impact on blood sugar and is safe for diabetics. Stevia has also been used to remedy conditions such as dandruff, gingivitis, and digestive upset.

Clearing bad habits from your life is no easy task, but that is certainly not to say it is impossible. I guarantee there are few greater feelings than accepting a challenge, setting your goal, and achieving it. Knowing that you have control over your health and the direction it takes is the ultimate in empowerment. Replacing bad habits with good ones is the first great step in that direction.

UNDIET LIVING

UnDiet for Abundance Mantra

Crunch on carrots, not on candy.

Make Love in the Kitchen

Just a little taste is not fine.

- Cheat days don't exist when you're creating delicious new habits.
- If you want something sweet, make it yourself.
- Ignore the games your mind plays that tells you it's the last time. The last time has passed.
- Steer clear of the places, peeps, and things that will derail your will power.

TRANSITIONAL TIPS AND TRICKS TO MAKE IT HAPPEN

Break those habits.

Choose three goals you want to achieve and identify the three (or more) habits that are keeping you from getting those going on. Use the steps provided to set yourself up for super success in establishing new and great habits.

No more refined sugar.

Going cold turkey on this one. If there is sugar on the label you are over it. Instead choose whole, healthier sweetener options. No more refined sugar.

Dig into the emotions, not the ice cream.

Bringing a level of consciousness to what fuels your habits and cravings will be the first step in eliminating them. Get help when you need it. Getting to the root motivator for the habit is what will lead to lasting success.

Catch you later, caffeine.

Ease yourself off coffee slowly, perhaps by drinking as frequently but in smaller cups, replacing every other cup with a cup of herbal tea, or avoiding the coffee places you enjoy most. Find what works and do it!

Build a team.

Choose a habit to break and a goal to achieve and bring together your support posse. Find someone to be accountable to who truly supports your goals.

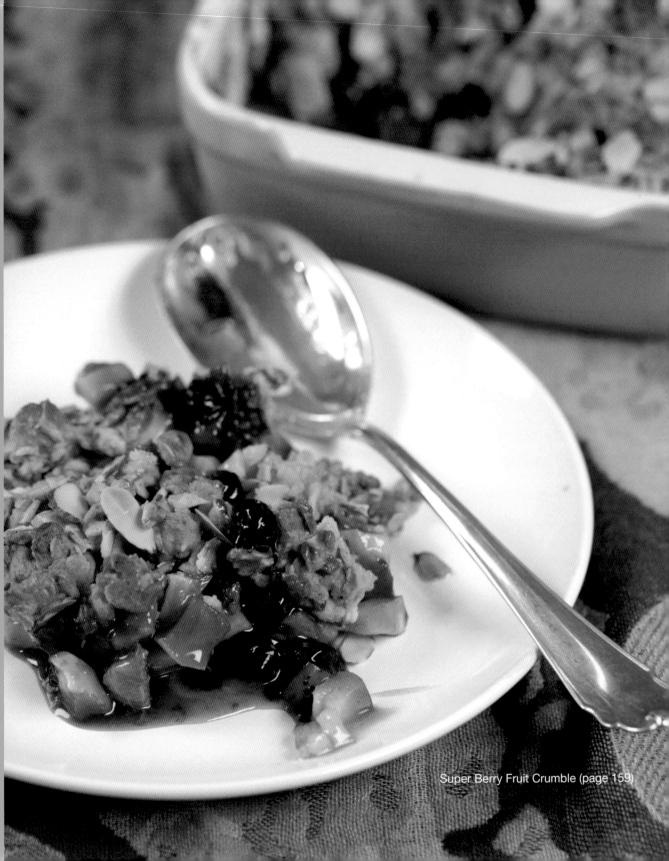

Super Berry Fruit Crumble (page 159)

Super Berry Fruit Crumble

Serves: 8

FRUIT BOTTOM

2 cups	blueberries	500 mL
2 cups	strawberries, quartered	500 mL
2 cups	apple, cut into ½-inch (1.5-cm) cubes	500 mL
½ cup	raw honey	125 mL
1 tbsp	arrowroot starch	15 mL

CRUMBLE TOPPING

⅔ cup	brown rice flour	150 mL
⅔ cup	rolled oats	150 mL
½ cup	sliced or slivered almonds	125 mL
½ cup	raw honey	125 mL
¼ cup	coconut oil	50 mL
¾ tsp	cinnamon	4 mL
½ tsp	allspice	2 mL

DIRECTIONS

- Preheat oven to 350°F (180°C).
- Mix fruit, raw honey and arrowroot, and spread into an 11- x 9-inch (2.5 L) glass baking dish. Flatten mixture with a spatula making sure it is evenly spread.
- In a medium mixing bowl, combine all topping ingredients, then crumble evenly over fruit mixture. If fruit doesn't look completely covered, add additional flour, almonds, or oats until surface is covered.
- Bake for 45 minutes, or until lightly browned and bubbling.

Mix and Match Your Fruit!

Get experimental with whatever fruit is in season. Here are some great combinations:

APPLE CRANBERRY

5 cups (1.25 L) apples and 1 cup (250 mL) fresh or dried cranberries.

STRAWBERRY RHUBARB

3 cups (750 mL) each.

PEACH

6 cups (1.5 L) peaches, sliced.

SUMMER BERRY

2 cups (500 mL) each strawberries, blueberries, and raspberries.

Spiced Apple-Carrot Cake or Muffins

Makes: 12 muffins

DRY INGREDIENTS

¾ cup	brown rice flour	175 mL
¾ cup	buckwheat flour	175 mL
½ cup	ground almonds	125 mL
1 tsp	baking powder	5 mL
1 tsp	baking soda	5 mL
1 tsp	cinnamon	5 mL
¼ tsp	nutmeg	1 mL
¼ tsp	allspice	1 mL
½ tsp	sea salt	2 mL

WET INGREDIENTS

⅓ cup	maple syrup	75 mL
⅓ cup	raw honey	75 mL
¼ cup	coconut oil, softened	50 mL
1	organic egg or 1 serving of chia paste (see page 87)	1
⅓ cup	applesauce	75 mL
⅓ cup	coconut milk or water	75 mL
1 tbsp	apple cider vinegar	15 mL
1 tsp	vanilla extract	5 mL
1 cup	carrot, grated	250 mL
1 cup	apple, cut into ½-inch (1.5-cm) cubes	250 mL

DIRECTIONS

- Preheat oven to 350°F (180°C).
- Grease cake pan or muffin tin with coconut oil and dust with brown rice flour.
- In large bowl, mix all dry ingredients together.
- In a separate bowl, mix together wet ingredients, and add to dry ingredients. Stir until smooth.
- Add carrots and apples, and stir until just mixed. Don't go overboard – you want the baking powder and baking soda to do rising magic in the oven, not in your mixing bowl.
- Pour batter into greased cake pan or muffin tin.
- For cake: bake for 35–40 minutes, or until a toothpick inserted into the middle of the cake comes out clean.
- For muffins: bake for 30–35 minutes, or until a toothpick inserted into the middle of the muffin comes out clean.
- Allow to cool for 10–15 minutes, then transfer to a cooling rack.

Batch Prep: Have on hand for fresh-baked goodies!

Combine 3 cups (750 mL) each of brown rice flour and buckwheat flour, 2 cups (500 mL) ground almonds, 1 tbsp (15 mL) each of baking powder and baking soda, and ½ tsp (2 mL) sea salt. This recipe would need 2 cups (500 mL) and 1 tbsp (15 mL) of mix.

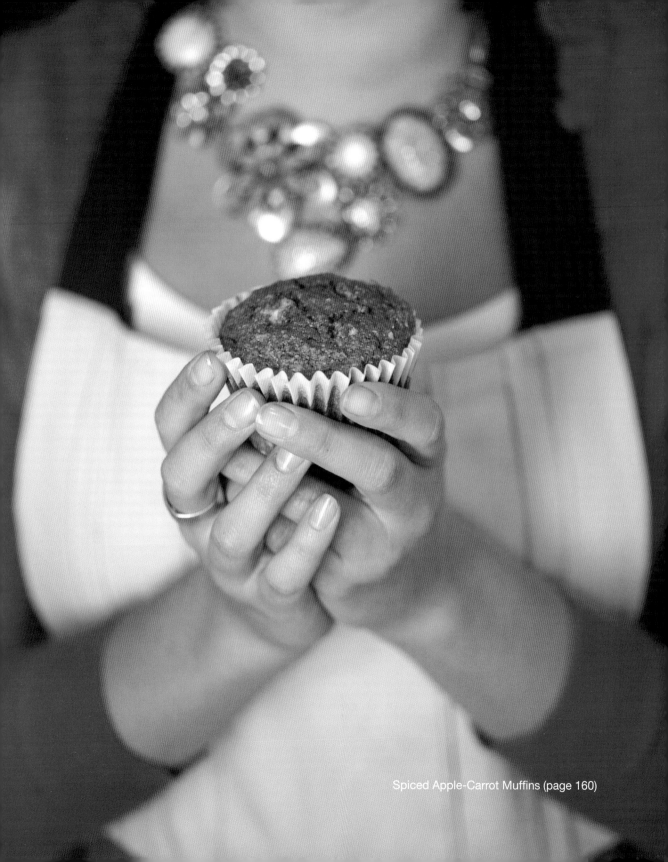

Spiced Apple-Carrot Muffins (page 160)

Almond Power Cookies

Makes: 12 cookies

1½ cups	ground almonds	375 mL
½ cup	pecans, finely chopped	125 mL
⅓ cup	shredded dried coconut	75 mL
¼ cup	maple syrup	50 mL
¼ cup	coconut oil	50 mL
¼ cup	dried cranberries (optional)	50 mL
¼ cup	dairy-free chocolate chips or cacao nibs (optional)	50 mL
	pinch of sea salt	

DIRECTIONS

- Preheat oven to 350°F (180°C).
- Mix all ingredients together.
- Take about 2 tablespoons of dough, roll into a ball, and then flatten on parchment-lined baking sheet.
- Bake until aromatic and slightly browned at the edges, about 20 minutes.
- Transfer to cooling rack. They will crisp up as they cool.

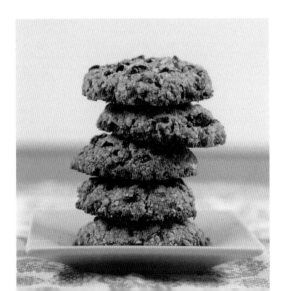

Banana Chocolate Soft Serve

Serves: 6

14 oz	full-fat organic coconut milk	400 mL
¼ cup	raw honey	50 mL
1	large banana	1
2 tsp	lemon juice	10 mL
3 tbsp	dried coconut, raw or roasted	45 mL
⅓ cup	cocoa powder	75 mL

DIRECTIONS

- Put all ingredients into the blender and blend until smooth.
- Reserve ⅓ cup (75 ml) of mixture in a mason jar and store in the fridge; pour the remaining mix into one or two ice cube trays and freeze.
- To serve: in a food processor, blend together frozen ice-cream cubes and reserved unfrozen mixture until smooth and creamy.
- Serve immediately.

Blueberry Bubbly

Serves: 2

1 cup	100 percent pure blueberry juice	250 mL
1 cup	soda water	250 mL
2	lemon or lime wedges	2
	ice cubes (optional)	

DIRECTIONS

- In a medium pitcher or jar, mix together the blueberry juice and soda water.
- Pour 1 cup (250 mL) of mix into each glass. Add ice if desired.
- Garnish with lemon or lime wedge and serve.

> Mix this cocktail up with any of your favorite fresh-pressed juices. Pure pomegranate also makes an amazing wine-replacing cocktail.

Easy Ginger Ale

Serves: 2

3 inches	fresh ginger root	8 cm
2 cups	soda water	500 mL
1 tbsp	raw honey or other natural sweetener	15 mL
2 tbsp	lemon juice (optional)	30 mL
	ice cubes or frozen grapes	

DIRECTIONS

- Drape a cheesecloth or nut sack over a bowl or jar, and grate ginger over top.
- Once fully grated, squeeze out juice.
- In a pitcher or jar, stir together ginger, soda water, sweetener, and lemon.
- Serve chilled with a few ice cubes or frozen grapes, and add a glass straw for a party in your glass.

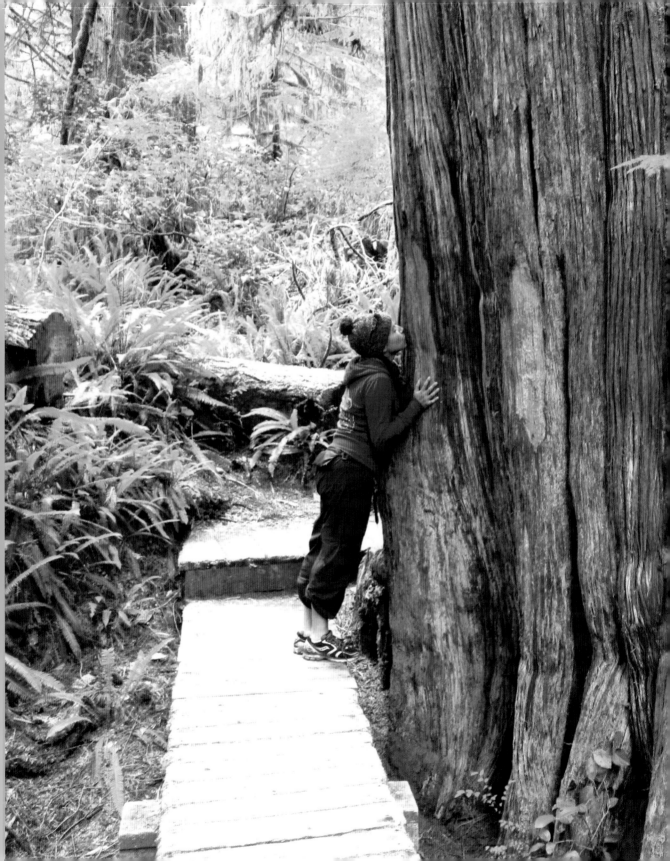

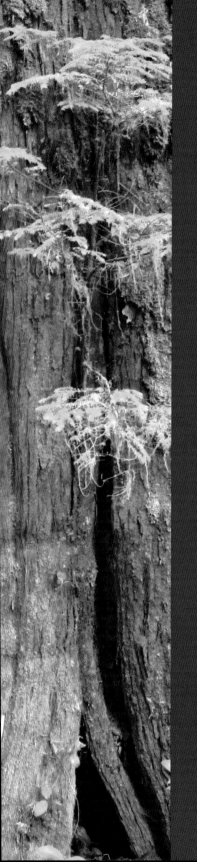

CHAPTER 8

There Is No "Away"

Remember that time in your life when all that was most important could be zipped into a slightly oversized backpack and carried with you hither and thither all over the globe? To be nineteen again, right? I would save up all year for my summer adventures – Europe, the Middle East, Australia, Fiji, Africa – all with my life packed on my back. Whether we're going camping, away for a weekend, or ten weeks living like a little explorative-bohemian-hobo-hippie, we know we can manage with much less than we have.

I wouldn't buy anything that wasn't an immediate need or consumable. I did my laundry once a week and all that I collected along the way were memories, love affairs, and tacky bracelets or anklets that I somehow thought made my appearance more legitimately bohemian, hobo, and hippie.

What I often noticed when I came home was that I had a re- ally hard time parting with my travel wardrobe and making friends again with everything else that was overflowing my closet – and all the other stuff that seemed to be cluttering up my life.

Years later, when I was diagnosed with Crohn's and moved to California for a few months to heal, I truly realized how little I actually needed and how unimportant most of my stuff was. Seems to me that the more experiences we collect, and the more we learn and grow, the less we need to carry with us, whether it be physical stuff or poundage on the booty.

What does any of this have to do with UnDieting to vibrant health? It has everything to do with the UnDiet revolution because we're learning to break some rules. We think we need to buy all these fancy-shmancy processed foods with these high and mighty health claims to be living the good life – and to live the good life means doing so as cheaply and conveniently as possible. The Un-Diet is about simplifying. It's about cutting out extra steps, middle people, and overpackaging. It's about cleaning out the clutter and getting the biggest bang for every cent and every bite we take out of this world, starting with our food. In this chapter we're going to trash talk – or rather, talk about trash. We're going to learn about how to batch cook to reduce what we toss and save money in the process, and I will convince you, I am quite sure, that we need to be buying more in bulk – more whole and unprocessed ingredients to improve our health and reduce the waste we make.

This does not mean that you have to grow your hair long, wear a flowing skirt, cover yourself in bohemian-hobo-hippie beads, put your arms around each other, and sing "Kumbaya" (though that could be fun with a guitar and a sky full of stars on a warm summer's night). This is about waking right on up to what's going on out there. Can I get a "Hey now"? Hey now!

THE FOOD WASTE WE MAKE

I will never forget my very first trip to a garbage dump. I was about eight years old and my family lived in Winnipeg, Manitoba, at the time. One summer weekend, our next-door neighbors, the Haracks, invited me up to their cottage at Royal Lake, a couple of hours outside Winnipeg. At around dusk, Brian, the dad, suggested we head over to the dump to drop off some trash and see if we could spot any bears.

We drove up and unloaded our contribution to the heap. The smell of a garbage dump at the end of a hot summer's day is something special. I had

never smelled anything like that; an odor that is like rank blue cheese thrown into a blender with some flat orange soda: sickeningly sour and sweet, complemented by the lingering heat of the day. I had never fathomed a place like this before. Why would I? Eight-year-old me knew that I was to put trash in the bin. I knew that once a week a truck came and took the trash away. I had never questioned where all that garbage was taken – and sadly, most people never do.

As we gazed out over the heap of waste, the piles and piles of stuff that people sent to the land we call "away," I saw the bears come over the garbage horizon. The vision of the trash heap being picked through by a family of bears has stuck with me.

A trip to the dump is now a regular occurrence to deposit the trash from my family cottage and I never fail to be astounded by the insane volume of needless garbage, with loads of it coming from the packaging of foods we shouldn't be consuming anyway.

I learned an important lesson early: there is no "away." When we throw something away, it has an address. It's usually a pit, just outside a city, and ideally just far enough away from any community that no one has to smell it, or develop tumors from the breakdown of the waste matter infiltrating the water system. But it is there, likely loaded with seagulls and rats picking at the things we mindlessly toss in the trash every single day thinking that by putting things into the garbage bin, and then taking that garbage bin to the curb for pick up, we have done our part by "cleaning up."

It's crazy to think that if everyone on the planet consumed and then created the waste that we do in North America, we'd need three to five

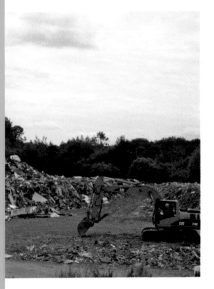

planets just to manage it all.[1] According to the Organization for Economic Co-operation and Development's (OECD) Environmental Data Compendium, in 2002 the United States led the way for garbage production with 1,675 pounds (760 kilograms) per person per year. Australia came in second with 1,524 pounds (690 kilograms) and Canada ranked fifth with 1,411 pounds (640 kilograms) per person per year.[2]

A lot of the garbage we're making comes in three very avoidable forms: paper, plastic, and food. The United States wastes the most food, which has an environmental impact globally. According to a report by the U.S. Environmental Protection Agency, the United States generates more than 34 million tons of food waste each year.[3] Holy shmizer! In Canada, it is estimated that 27 billion dollars worth of food ends up in landfills each year.[4] According to World Vision Canada, the residents in the city of Toronto alone toss out 16.5 million pounds (7.5 million kilograms) of food every month.[5]

Food waste is more than 14 percent of the total municipal solid waste. Even more shameful is that less than 3 percent of the 34 million tons of food waste created in 2009 was recovered and recycled. That means that 33 million tons were trucked off to the place we call "away."[6] Food waste now represents the single largest component of municipal landfills and incinerators in the United States. Following close behind, for your interest, are yard scraps (which could be reduced if we all just planted edible gardens) and plastic. In the average American home, each week 12 percent of meat, 16 percent of grains and nearly one quarter of fruits and vegetables are tossed out. The cost of that averages out to be over 43 billion dollars worth of household food waste annually.[7] *Oyegevuletshane!* As if that weren't bad enough, 18 percent of vegetables that are grown don't even make it to the stores before they perish.[8]

One of my colleagues, Lisa Borden, who shares her no-fuss, no-muss waste-reducing strategies later in this chapter, often invokes the ancient African proverb: "If you think you're too small to make a difference, try sleeping in a room with a mosquito." Even the littlest of changes that you weren't doing yesterday can have a massive impact over the long run. If you pick up a coffee or tea every day on your way to work and drink it from a paper cup, with an extra paper band around it, you're tossing at least 260 paper cups annually. If you use paper napkins at your meals at home and out, you're throwing away roughly a thousand or more napkins a year. Just you! What about the rest of your family? If you throw out celery and carrots every week because you were too lazy to prep and eat them, you may think it's no biggie. But what if everyone on your street also did that? You get where I'm going here?

Low-impact living doesn't have to mean the revamp of your whole wide world. It does, however, need a wee bit of awareness regarding your habits and taking a look at the little things you can start to make shipshape, which will benefit your health, your bank account, and the planet. That means you can start to save up to visit the Amazon rainforests, swim in the deep blue seas, drink spring water from some far-off waterfalls, and also eat fresh herbs from your very own window or backyard garden. All this because you did some wee powerful stuff to make sure these things remain available.

"*Every aspect of our lives is, in a sense, a vote for the kind of world we want to live in.*"
– Frances Moore Lappe

A LESSON ON PLASTIC

Recycling helps. A little bit. Recycling plastic drinking bottles, tin cans, paper boxes from our crackers, and glass jars from our honey is a good step. Wouldn't a better step be to not need to have to recycle so much? I think we forget that there is an order to the recycling mantra of "Reduce, Reuse, Recycle." Notice that *reduce* and *reuse* come well before *recycle*.

Whether we recycle it or not, once a piece of plastic is created, it is with us forever. Every piece of plastic ever created on this planet since plastic started being created still remains in one form or another. According to Worldwatch Institute's State of the World 2004 report, "an estimated four to five trillion plastic bags – including large trash bags, thick shopping bags, and thin grocery bags – were produced globally in 2002. Roughly 80 percent of those bags were used in North America and Western Europe. Every year, Americans reportedly throw away 100 billion plastic grocery bags, which can clog drains, crowd landfills, and leave an unsightly blot on the landscape."[9] About a thousand miles west of San Francisco is the Great Pacific Garbage Patch (also called the Pacific Trash Vortex), a heaping floating mass of plastic debris twice the size of Texas. Blech!

Plastic is not just in the obvious things like water bottles, bags, and hummus containers, but it also lines our tin cans, is in our shower curtains, and unless it's packaged in unlined paper or glass with a glass lid, it has likely made contact with every packaged food item in our home. We are coming into contact with and producing too much plastic garbage.

Like pharmaceutical medications, plastic has become an easy go-to solution, chosen most often for convenience, not necessity. When we really need to use plastic, we can; however, there are other options for our day-to-day lives that can help us to reduce our consumption and use of it. Think about this. What if you had to go a whole week, no wait, let's just go a whole day, trying to consume or use things that have had no contact with plastic? I wish you luck – it's tough, nearly impossible.

A little bit here and there is not the end of the world. A lot here and there will be, though. In terms of our health, there are oodles of reasons we might want to avoid foods that come in, are heated in, or hang out for a long time in plastic. Ready for this?

WE'RE NOT IN THE 1950s ANYMORE – THE TUPPERWARE PARTY IS OVER

Flip over your fave food-storage container. What do you see? If you find the numbers 3 or 7, these sweet tubs of storage are now going to be used for your hair accessories or spare buttons and sewing supplies, not for food.

What's Behind Door Number 3?

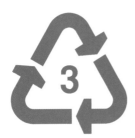

Number 3 is for polyvinyl chloride (PVC), also known as vinyl. When I was in high school, I was the student designer for my school fashion show and made my dear friend Vanessa, now an environmental journalist and author, wear an entire outfit made from shiny black PVC. I feel a wee bit bad. PVC has the sweet nickname of "the toxic plastic" for the presence of DEHA – a plastic softener that makes it the ideal material for really tight, shiny pants, inflatable palm trees, and malleable plastic wrap.

Exposure to this chemical can reduce bone mass, increase estrogen levels (thereby shrinking up the testicles of our fave teste owners), damage the liver (a vital organ for detoxing), and ultimately can be a contributing factor to the development of cancer. Adding insult to the horrid injury, production (and later deconstruction) of PVC releases carcinogenic dioxins into the environment and subsequently, into our dinner.[10] Don't panic – *yet!* PVC is not the most common plastic used for food-storage containers, but is often used to improve strength, flexibility, and stickiness (what the companies call "performance") in plastic wrap.

What's Behind Door Number 7?

Number 7 includes a whole buffet of several plastics – miscellaneous plastics that don't fit into the other categories. This plastic is comprised mostly of polycarbonate. The who of the what? Polycarbonate, something you may have never heard of, contains within its chemical cocktail something called bisphenol A or BPA, something you probably have heard of for the rage against the machine it caused when mommas found out it was in baby bottles and teething toys. One of its prime damaging effects is on the reproductive system, not ideal for anyone, especially for wee ones still developing. Essentially, BPA mimics our own hormones, estrogen to be precise (when they come from synthetic sources like plastic, we call them xenoestrogens), and has been linked to all kinds of sex hormone–related cancers such as prostate and breast cancers. Additionally, it can contribute to early onset of puberty and reproductive-organ defects, such as smaller-than-normal junk in men. Since the 1960s, sperm counts have been cut in half and "rates of testicular cancer have doubled in the last 20 years."[11]

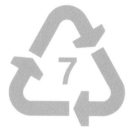

The U.S. Food and Drug Administration admits that these bad guys can leach into our food from the containers they were stored in, but it hangs on to the claim that there are safe levels.[12] One of the most common sources of BPA in the adult diet is canned food. BPA is used in the liners of tin cans to help preserve the food inside – the problem is that this chemical leaches into the food and then we eat it right up. Plastic use has never been higher, and the most common forms of cancer are breast and prostate.[13] I am pretty sure it's safe to assume we all know someone who has dealt with ovarian, breast, prostate, or testicular cancer. Could there be a connection? Better safe than sorry goes a long way here.

Some of us may be totally freaking out and ready to trash anything and everything that has rubbed up against a little plastic. There are, however,

Bye-bye, BPA: Many companies have made great effort and put out extra expense to ensure they're not using BPA–lined cans for their products. Read the label, and choose the BPA–free option.

some easy ways to cut way back on our love affair with plastic both in and out of the kitchen.

A FEW WAYS TO SEVER THE TOXIC PLASTIC TIES

❀ **Leave the petroleum for your car.** I am pretty sure everything can be stored in mason jars. My fridge is proof. Instead of mixing petroleum, which is where plastic comes from, with your food, look for alternatives, such as glass, stoneware, ceramic, and stainless steel.

❀ **Get up close and personal with plastic.** All plastics are marked with an identification coding system. This is the number surrounded by arrows.

1 polyethylene terephthalate (PETE)

2 high-density polyethylene (HDPE)

3 vinyl, polyvinyl chloride (PVC)

4 low-density polyethylene (LDPE)

5 polypropylene (PP)

6 polystyrene (PS)

7 other (includes polycarbonate, acrylic, polylactic acid, fiberglass)

This means that when you do need to use plastics, there are some options that are better than others. Stick with those numbered 1, 2, 4, and 5 — and just try to use them minimally.

❀ **Time for retirement.** We hate to throw this stuff out. I know. But sometimes it's just the better choice. If your containers are really worn out, scratched, or show deep stains (tomatoes are a common culprit), this would be a good sign that this baby is leaching and no longer serving our health. As the plastics get used and abused, they do begin to break down, shedding their wear and tear into our food. Find a different use, recycle it or, if you can't do either, it's time to toss.

✽ **If you can't take the heat . . .** Never, ever put hot food or reheat food in a plastic container, especially any food containing fat. As we now know, toxins love to make a nest in the fat cells of the body. Fat cells in our food are also prime locales for these toxins to jump from our container and sail the seas of fat into our bodies.

✽ **Plastic + microwave = toxic lunch.** I am hoping at this point, if you haven't replaced your microwave with a juicer, that you've at least replaced it with a stereo system or duct taped the door shut. When something is "micro-wave safe," it means it won't melt or explode – but it doesn't mean it won't leach chemicals into your food. Have you ever smelled burning plastic? Toxic, right? Heat at any level commences this off-gas of horribleness into your dinner. Put your food in oven-safe glass and heat it in the oven or heat it up on the stove in a pan. It's worth the tiny bit of extra time.

✽ **Don't taint your sandwich.** No need to wrap food in plastic wrap. Seriously. There are re-usable options.

HOW TO TAKE OUT WITHOUT
BY LISA BORDEN

Everything we consume creates some amount of waste. Even more impor-tant than recycling is reducing, refusing, and reusing. Recycling is not justifi-cation to use something; it's just a last resort for the stuff you *have* to use.

Americans toss out enough paper bags and plastic cups and cutlery every year to circle the equator 300 times.[14] Since this waste and other pack-aging can remain in our landfills forever, and the plastics could in fact be poisoning us all, let's jump to the conclusion that these single-use dispos-ables are not convenient.

Say NO to unnecessary packaging and tote around your own plastic-free reusables, such as:

✽ **Lunch bags.** If it's insulated, make sure that it's lead-free.
✽ **Glass or stainless steel food containers.** Leak-proof ones are a huge plus.

❀ **Insulated mugs.** To keep your hot drinks hot and your cold drinks cold.

❀ **Plastic-free reusable water bottle.** Perspective: if you leave your wallet at home, you can't buy anything; if you leave your water bottle at home, you can't buy bottled water. Get a glass and a tap and drink.

❀ **Organic cloth napkin or three.** You have to do laundry anyway, right?

❀ **Stainless steel or bamboo cutlery and glass drinking straws.** Easy to wash and stash.

So, stop throwing your money away – literally – on disposables and over-packaged foods. Enjoy your food, save your money, improve your health, and help our planet by embracing the Bring Your Own (BYO) revolution.

Lisa Borden, owner of Borden Communications, takes a unique approach to holistically marketing eco-intelligent living and working. Some of her favorite titles are: catalyst for change, enthusiastic philanthropist, inspiration agent, strategist, mother of three, and wannabe organic farmer.

PACKAGE-FREE MEANS WHOLE AND (MOST OFTEN) HEALTHY

Do you know that if you follow the UnDiet rule-breaking philosophy, your lifestyle automatically drops down on the waste factor? For lack of a better cliché, if we're not part of the problem then we're part of the solution. By eating whole, unprocessed foods, and doing so with all your reusable containers, you dramatically reduce what lands in the garbage. You shed the negative impact and double dose on the positive goodness. That is low-impact living.

One of the easiest ways to follow along with the UnDiet tips and tricks is just to ditch the packaged food. You be quiet. I hear you rolling on the floor laughing. I hear you! I know you don't have nineteen hours a day to spend in the kitchen grinding grains, watching dough rise, and baking the loaf from scratch. We've established already that we are all busy bees. But since we've already gone through all the reasons why we should be keener watchdogs when it comes to reading labels, we know there are many tricky ingredients hiding inside, wrapped in a heap of toxic plastic. I don't know about you, but I plan to stick around for a while and would like my health and the planet to join me.

When we shed the packaged foods, we shed a lot of the nutrient-depleted junk because now most of the processing is happening in our own kitchens. A head of broccoli doesn't come in a package. Neither do apples. You can also choose to buy your salad greens loosey-goosey rather than dry-cleaned and plastic packaged. It is now time that I fully break down for you what all this whole-food chitter-chatter is about as we explore some of the foundational plant-based foods we are growing to know and love to bits.

Whole Grains and Whole-Grain Flours

Did you know there are more grains out there than just wheat? Did you also know that wheat is one of the first foods I recommend peeps stay away from if they have any kind of health problems? It's in abso-freaking-lutely everything.

Here is a little science lesson we should have received in school when we were too busy learning about the ever practical and useful lessons of obtuse angles and logarithms. A grain is considered whole when all three parts — the bran, the germ, and the cutely named endosperm (no relation to the other kind of sperm) — are present. We all know that fruits and veggies contain beneficial fiber, antioxidants, vitamins, and minerals, but rarely do we think about the goodness in the whole grain. Most of the fiber, antioxidants, and mineral and vitamin magic of grains is found in the germ and the bran; the first bits to be removed when a whole kernel of wheat gets transformed in the ooey, gooey, sticky starch that makes up our fluffy white colon-clogging bagels. Our government-regulated food guides might say that a bagel and a bowl of whole rolled oats porridge count equally as a serving. They may be equal in calories, but definitely not in nutrition.

detailed preparaton directions are online visit http://bit.ly/UnDiet to download your copy

We burn up to 50 percent more calories when the processing of our whole foods happens inside our body. Turning whole foods into refined or processed foods requires energy. Another name for that is calories. When those calories are used up in the factories, by the time the foods enter our body, most of the work has been done. When we eat the whole-food version, our body does the work. This helps us to burn more calories per bite of whole food simply in the metabolic process.[15]

More Beans,
Fewer Farts:
Soak the beans for
four to six hours; rinse
thoroughly. Bring them to
a boil in a saucepan of
water, drain, rinse again,
then cook. Cooking
beans with fennel, ginger,
garlic, and sea vegeta-
bles like kelp and kombu
also helps. Lastly, eat
small amounts of beans
and lentils regularly to
help your body adjust.

detailed preparaton
directions are online
visit http://bit.ly/UnDiet
to download your copy

Lentils and Beans

Beans, beans, good for the heart, the more we eat them the more we . . . Yes, I have now stooped to that level to get you on side with the need for beans and lentils in the UnDiet. These little hard pellets of nutrition are too often ignored, but we need them so much. Often used in traditional Indian, West Indian, and Middle Eastern cooking, lentils and beans benefit pretty much everyone, unless suffering from intense digestive challenges.

Why do beans make us toot? Beans have chains of sugars in them that are tough for the body to fully digest. When these undigested sugars make their way into our lower intestinal region, the little naturally occurring bacteria have a hey-day chow-down and mow down on those sugars like it's an all-you-can-eat boooofaye (that's Meghan for buffet). These bacteria release gas, which is what we toot out. Lentils and beans are low glycemic, which makes them great for managing blood sugar levels, fueling the health of the heart, helping us look young and sprightly, and loading us with fiber to keep our bowels in fine form. They have tons of complex carbohydrates to fuel us; essential fatty acids to keep our brain, nervous system, and endocrine system running like a well-oiled machine; and, of course, protein to maintain healthy hair, skin, tissues, and blood.

The nutrients in lentils and beans are released into the body slowly, so an added bonus is that when we eat them, we feel pretty darn satiated for an extended period of time.

Nuts and Seeds

I am not talking about peanuts or tinned mixes of salt with a side of hydrogenated oil-fried nuts, or anything beer battered, or whatever that mess is they put on the nuts over at the local pub and your favorite airline. We're talking whole, raw, and organic nuts and seeds, eaten in moderation. These potent gems of nutritious loving are packed to the shell with nutrients. Most of all, they are high in all those über-awesometown fats.

Let's take a moment and think about seeds. Seeds are what starts it all. They are nature's way of making life happen. Imagine how much nutritional power they have! Seeds are small but mighty capsules that house the massive abundance of nutrients that will grow and nourish a brand-shiny-new plant.

These nuggets of golden health can be used as snacks, but they can also be turned into butters, made into milks (see page 56), or ground into flours for baking, breading, and stuffing needs.

detailed preparaton directions are online visit http://bit.ly/UnDiet to download your copy

With their gold mine of healthy minerals and their niacin and folic-acid contents, seeds are an excellent nutrition package. They are among the better plant sources of iron and zinc. In fact, one ounce of pumpkin seeds contains almost twice as much iron as three ounces of skinless chicken breast. [16]

MAKING IT FROM SCRATCH

Don't go thinking you need to change your name to Holly Homemaker just yet, though it does have a bit of a ring to it. Making things from scratch doesn't mean you have to trade in your career, your hobbies, or your designer pumps. It's simply looking at the things you most often buy in packages and making a squeak of time in your schedule once or twice a month to easily make a few batches from scratch. This not only cuts down on the garbage we make, but also on the cost, all while multiplying the health-promoting benefits. When we cook from scratch in our own kitchen, there is no filler goo in the food, no unnamed flours, no processed oils, and no artificial preservatives. Every bite is pure power, even when it's a treat.

The very best approach to tackle this whole from-scratch thing is to first take on some skills and secrets in the batch-cooking department. Take some time to get the staples ready and you'll always be ready and set to go.

BATCH COOKING TIPS TO GET YOU ROCKING PACKAGE-FREE AND LOW IMPACT

Soups and Stews

❋ Make a few at one time. Once you are chopping, slicing, simmering, and pureeing, pick a couple of soups to make. Make the mess all at once so there's less to clean up later.

❀ Allow your soups to cool and transfer to half-quart (500 mL) mason jars for single servings or 1-quart (1-liter) mason jars for two. Store one or two in the fridge for up to a week and freeze the rest. Remember to leave about 2 inches (5 cm) of room at the top of the jar to avoid cracking in the freezing process.

❀ Don't worry if you don't have any stock on hand. Just add some extra veggies and sea salt to your soup instead of packaged or powdered stock.

❀ If taking it to work for lunch, allow it to defrost overnight in the sink, heat up in a pot on the stove, transfer to a thermos, and you are good to go.

❀ If getting ready for dinner, take it out in the morning and it will be ready to rock by the time you get home.

Dips, Sauces, and Dressings

❀ Make one or two different sauces or dressings each week.

❀ Store in half-pint (250 ml) mason jars in the fridge. Keep one jar of salad dressing or dip at home and take another to work.

❀ Extra pesto, sauces, and dips can be frozen in small jars or in ice-cube trays so that you have an easy single serving at the ready.

Veggie Prep

❀ Don't be lazy! Make veggie prep part of your batch-cooking routine.

❀ Buy your vegetables fresh, cut and prep them, then freeze any extras in airtight containers.

Burgers and Patties

Why buy processed versions? Just do it yourself, for goodness sake, and fill them up to the brim with veggies.

❀ Mix your ingredients, cook them as directed, allow to cool, place on a wax-paper- or parchment-lined cookie sheet, and stick in the freezer. When frozen, transfer to an airtight container.

❀ Take out what you need when you need it. Defrost on your counter and then place in a preheated oven at around 250–300°F (120–150°C) for about fifteen minutes, just until heated. You can, of course, put them in frozen, but they will take a little longer to heat up.

Crackers and Cereal

Crackers and cereal are likely the worst culprits of the packaged-food world, but it's also the easiest category to make from scratch. You can make massive batches, and, if stored in an airtight container, they will last as long as you want.

* Pick one or two dry cereal or granola recipes. Mix, bake, cool, store in airtight glass jars.

* For mixed muesli or cooked granola, combine all of the dry ingredients you like to use, and yes, this could even include small amounts of your favorite dry sweetener like Sucanat or palm sugar. When it's time to cook, just take out a measured scoop and cook away.

* Should any moisture creep in and they go limp, just put them back in the oven for a few moments to make them crispy again.

Beans, Lentils, and Grains

Best consumed fresh, however, given that whole grains take a little longer to cook, you might as well pick one or two that you're going to love for a few days and make a whole bunch.

* Use these prepped beans, grains, and lentils in your salads, soups, and stews. You can even add a few spoonfuls to your soups and stews before you freeze them.

* Store cooked beans, lentils, and grains in the fridge in a sealed container for three days and reheat by putting on the stove in a pot and adding a little water or oil to avoid sticking.

* If it looks like you made more than you're going to eat, freeze them.

Baked Goodness

A treat is a treat and should be treated as such. Cravings will come, and you're gonna want something. Make it yourself! If you have some of the good, homemade sweets on hand, you'll be better prepared to resist the temptation of the processed faux-treats made with white sugar, bad fats, and refined nutrient-deficient flours.

* Bake a batch of your fave treats one or two times a month.

* Store in airtight containers and take out just what you want when you want it.

* Reheat in your oven and it's like having something freshly baked every single time.

If baking your own crackers from scratch is still a little too renaissance for you, just make sure when you buy your crackers that there is no BHT mentioned on the box as a coating on the plastic lining, or in the ingredient list. You also want to aim for bulk cracker packaging, as opposed to the types that package three or four crackers together within the larger package. Reduce your impact by reducing the waste.

Freeze It!
Made the batter, but have no time to bake or space to freeze the finished product? Freezing cookie dough means you can always show up at a party with freshly baked cookies. That's how we make friends with our UnDiet UnSupporters and turn them into cheerleaders.

❀ Cookies: Bake a batch and freeze the rest. Take out one or two when you want. Home-baked is always better than store-bought.

❀ Fruit crisps: Prep and bake in single-serve ramekins and freeze. Warm and bake in the oven when you want one.

❀ Cakes: Cut up into pieces and freeze individually so you aren't tempted to eat the whole thing.

Something really cool happens when we embrace a healthy lifestyle as our goal. We begin to value experiences as our most important possessions, and shoes and handbags take a back seat. It becomes a natural, or dare I say, an organic transition to becoming more mindful of not only what we're consuming in terms of what we eat, but also in terms of external resources. The moral of the story: garbage does not go "away." In this case, out of sight should not mean out of mind. Remember this and UnDiet your way to changing things up.

You're with me now. I can feel it.

UNDIET LIVING

UnDiet for Abundance Mantra

There is no "away."

Make Love in the Kitchen

Refuse then reduce and reuse.

Reduce consumption of all packaged goods.

Make staple foods from scratch.

Be mindful of the plastic villains.

Take out without.

Batch cook to reduce food waste.

TRANSITIONAL TIPS AND TRICKS TO MAKE IT HAPPEN

Packing lunch.

With your batch cooking solutions and a commitment to reducing food waste, it is time to start taking your lunch and snacks with you. Save money, reduce garbage, and enjoy the health benefits.

Say farewell to the disposable life.

Invest now and save later. Start storing food in glass instead of plastic. Ditch the plastic wrap for sealable stainless steel or glass and bring on the reusable sandwich bags, tote bags, mugs, and napkins.

Do it from scratch.

Choose three items that you always buy in a package that you will now fully commit to always making from scratch. My humble suggestion might be one cereal, one soup or stock, and one ready-to-rock entrée such as stew or burgers.

Get back to basics.

We feel lighter with less. Make time to clean stuff out. Take old clothes, dishes, furniture, and knickknacks to a local charity or thrift store. Lighten the load in your home or work environment.

Reduce, reuse, recycle.

Challenge yourself and your family to reduce the amount of garbage being made by everyday living. This will alter what you buy and also what you do with the packaging once you're done.

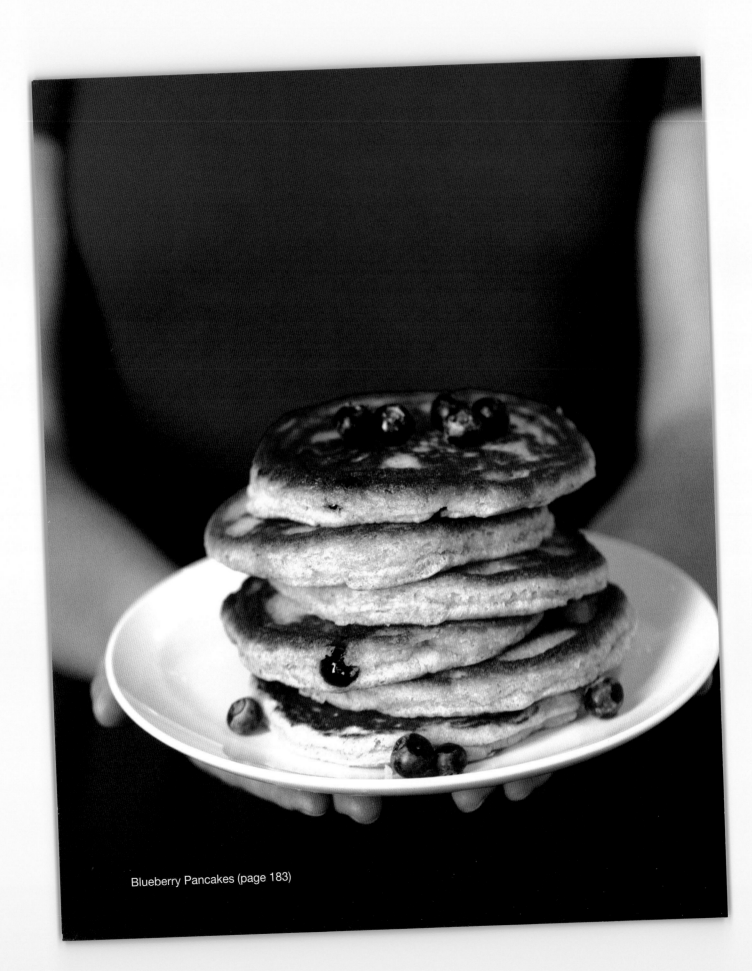

Blueberry Pancakes (page 183)

Blueberry Pancakes

Makes: 6 pancakes

PANCAKE MIX

2¼ cups	brown rice flour	550 mL
¾ cup	ground flaxseed	175 mL
1 tbsp	baking powder	15 mL
½ tsp	sea salt	2 mL
1 tbsp	cinnamon	15 mL

DIRECTIONS

- Mix ingredients.
- Store in a glass jar in your fridge or freezer for 4 months.

FRESH PANCAKES

1¼ cups	pancake mix	300 mL
¼ cup	applesauce	50 mL
2	organic eggs	2
1 tbsp	coconut oil, plus additional to coat pan	15 mL
2 tbsp	raw honey	30 mL
½ cup	almond milk (see page 56), or water	125 mL
1–2 cups	blueberries (if using frozen, do not thaw first)	250–500 mL

DIRECTIONS

- If you're making a whole bunch, preheat your oven to 200°F (100°C).
- In a large mixing bowl, combine applesauce, eggs, coconut oil, honey, and almond milk.
- Add the dry pancake mix to the wet ingredients and mix until smooth. Add blueberries and mix until evenly distributed.
- Heat the frying pan on high and melt 2 tsp coconut oil in the pan. Reduce heat to low-medium and spoon small dollops of batter in the pan and rotate in small circles to spread out.
- When you see bubbles, use a spatula to flip the pancake over. Resist the urge to turn the heat up too high.
- Transfer pancakes to an oven-safe dish, and place in the oven to keep warm until serving.

SUPER SYRUP

Equal parts each of:

Maple Syrup

Coconut oil

Flax oil

DIRECTIONS

- Add ingredients to a jar and shake.
- Pour over pancakes.
- Store any leftover syrup in the fridge.

My Favorite Granola

Serves: 8

2½ cups	rolled oats	625 mL
⅓ cup	buckwheat	75 mL
¼ cup	pumpkin seeds	50 mL
¼ cup	sunflower seeds	50 mL
¼ cup	slivered or coarsely chopped almonds	50 mL
¼ cup	shredded dried coconut	50 mL
1 tbsp	cinnamon	15 mL
¼ tsp	sea salt	1 mL
2 tbsp	coconut oil	30 mL
⅓ cup	raw honey	75 mL
¼ cup	organic dried cranberries or currants	50 mL

DIRECTIONS

- Preheat oven to 300°F (150°C).
- In a large mixing bowl, combine rolled oats, buckwheat, pumpkin seeds, sunflower seeds, almonds, coconut, cinnamon, and sea salt.
- In a small bowl, combine coconut oil and raw honey. Pour over dry mixture and stir well. Use your hands if you need to!
- Spread mix out on parchment-lined baking sheet and bake for 20 minutes.
- Stir around and bake for 20–30 minutes more or until light brown. Remove and let cool.
- Mix in cranberries and store in mason jars.

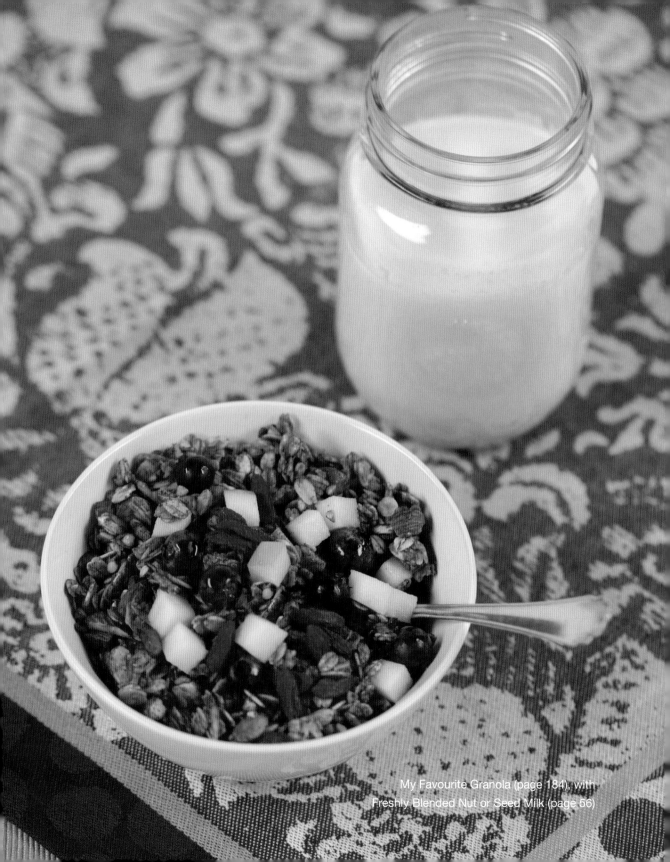

My Favourite Granola (page 184), with
Freshly Blended Nut or Seed Milk (page 56)

Sun-dried Tomato and Bean Hummus

Serves: 6

½ cup	organic, sulphite-free sun-dried tomatoes, soaked in water for a few hours (warm water speeds up the process)	125 mL
15 oz	can organic kidney beans, or 2 cups cooked	425 g
¼ cup	tahini (sesame paste)	50 mL
1	garlic clove, minced	1
1	ginger root, grated	1
2 tbsp	lemon juice	30 mL
2 tbsp	extra virgin olive oil	30 mL
1 tbsp	dried parsley	15 mL
1 tbsp	dried basil	15 mL
1 tbsp	dried oregano	15 mL
½ tsp	sea salt	2 mL
2 tbsp	water, or more if needed	30mL
	cayenne to taste	

DIRECTIONS

- Place all ingredients in your high-speed blender or food processor and process until smooth.
- Add water until desired consistency is reached. For more flavor, use the water you soaked the tomatoes in.

Herbed Quinoa Sesame Crackers

1⅓ cups	cup sesame seeds, ground	325 mL
¾ cup	flax seeds, ground	175 mL
2 tbsp	chia seeds, ground	30 mL
2 cups	cooked quinoa	500 mL
2 tsp	dried rosemary	10 mL
2 tsp	dried thyme	10 mL
2 tsp	dried oregano	10 mL
2 tsp	sea salt	10 mL
2 tbsp	water	30 mL

DIRECTIONS

- Preheat oven to 350°F (180°C).
- Grind seeds in a coffee grinder.
- In your food processor, process quinoa until relatively smooth and dough-like.
- Add ground seeds, herbs, and sea salt, and process. Add water 1 tbsp at a time if needed.
- Remove dough from food processor and place between two sheets of parchment paper. Roll it out until it's ⅛-inch thick. The thinner the dough, the crispier the crackers.
- Transfer parchment paper and dough to a cookie sheet and remove top layer of paper. Using a knife or cookie cutter, cut dough into desired shapes.
- Bake for 20 minutes, or until surfaces are firm and dry. Flip each over with a spatula and bake for another 10–15 minutes. Remove from oven and let cool.
- Store in an airtight container for upto a week, or in the fridge, or freeze for two months.

Meghan's No-Longer-Secret Tomato Sauce

Serves: 6–8

12	large tomatoes, de-seeded and pureed in a blender or food processor	12
1	onion, chopped	1
4	garlic cloves, minced	4
2	red peppers, coarsely chopped	2
2 cups	broccoli, coarsely chopped	500 mL
1 cup	purple cabbage, coarsely chopped	250 mL
4 cups	spinach, coarsely chopped	1 L
1 cup	shiitake mushrooms, coarsely chopped	250 mL
1 cup	fresh basil, coarsely chopped	250 mL
¼ cup	fresh parsley, coarsely chopped	50 mL
2 tbsp	raw honey	30 mL
1 tbsp	dried oregano	15 mL
1 tbsp	sea salt	15 mL
2 tsp	dried thyme	10 mL
½ tsp	cinnamon	2 mL
	zest of 1 lemon	
	pinch of nutmeg	
	cayenne to taste	
1 tbsp	arrowroot starch (optional)	15 mL

DIRECTIONS

- Put all the ingredients in a large, heavy-bottom, non-leaching saucepan, cover, and simmer for 35 minutes.

- Remove lid and simmer for another 20 minutes or until desired thickness is achieved, stirring occasionally. If you want to speed up the thickening process, remove 1 cup (250 mL) of liquid and blend with 1 tbsp (15 mL) arrowroot starch. Add this mixture back into the saucepan and stir well.

- Allow to cool completely. Store in glass jars or containers. If freezing, leave about 2 inches (5 cm) of space at the top of the jar.

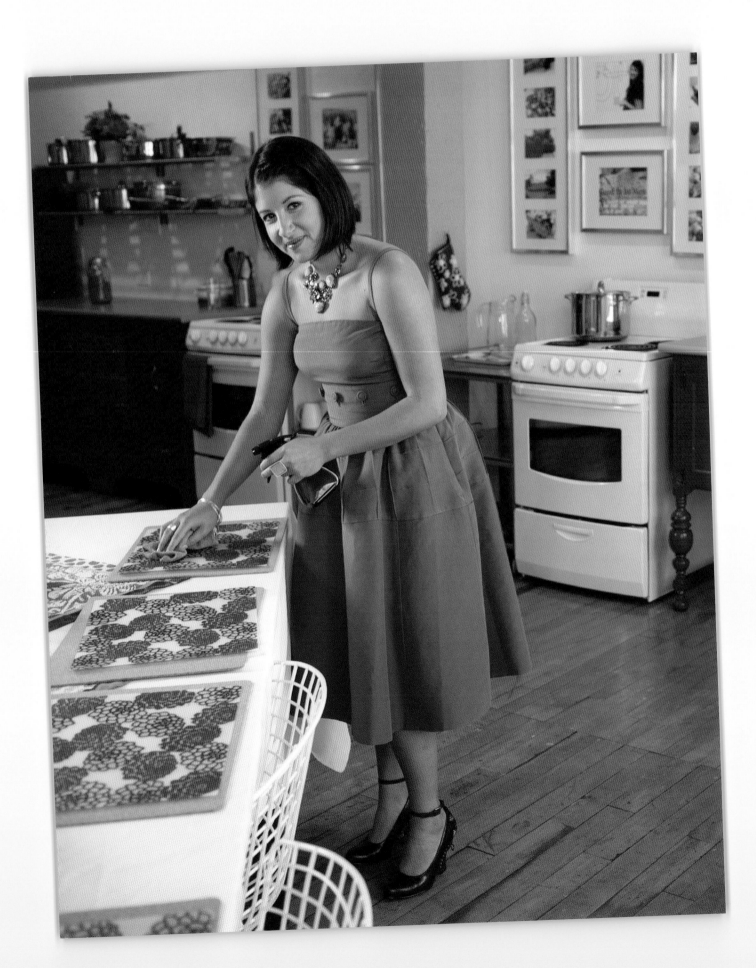

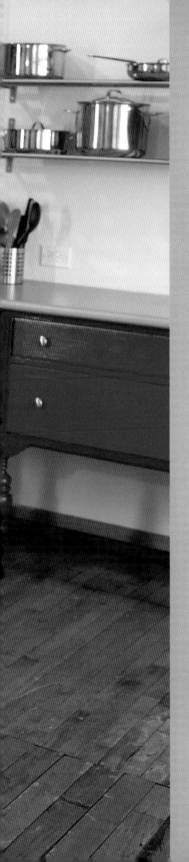

CHAPTER 9

A Touch of au Naturel

EDIBLE BEAUTY AND HOME CARE

Please tell me I am not the only young woman in love who has hung on to that article of clothing belonging to the object of my affection during a time apart? For me it was a mustard yellow T-shirt emblazoned with a sports team's logo. It belonged to my then-boyfriend Alexis. At twenty-one and head over heels, I decided to leave my boyfriend behind and carry on with my plans to spend the summer traveling with some girlfriends. I took his yellow T-shirt with me. I wouldn't wear the shirt. No, then it would have to be washed. I wanted to keep it just as it was for the whole two months I was away – smelling just like him or, rather, his cologne.

Two months later, the shirt still smelled of his cologne, as if he had only just taken it off. At the time, I failed to realize how wrong this actually was (both the smelling like cologne and the traveling with his shirt). I never thought to wonder how a shirt that was packed and unpacked, laid up against other clothing items, and transported thousands of miles, never lost one bit of its fragrance in that span of time. I never considered the toxic chemicals that made that happen.

On that note, it is time we do a little UnDiet making over on the old beauty routine. Have you ever given thought to what makes your vanilla moisturizer smell like vanilla? Or your lemon floor cleaner smell like lemons? Chances are it's neither vanilla beans nor fresh lemon juice. These extras, the things we smear on our body every day and inhale in the air, are all part of the cocktail that contributes to our health. It's time we cleanse out a little of that toxic clutter that's taking away from our natural inside-out glow. Time to explore the foods that make us shine with health, as well as taking a closer look at the goo we keep rubbing into our skin and painting our faces with. We have to.

NO NEED TO CRACK OPEN THE PATCHOULI OIL – YET

Consider this: if things are dirty and grubby and toxic on the inside, that ooey toxicity is going to want to come out. The internal waste becomes external in a few ways. Our skin is the largest organ of the body and is commonly referred to as the third kidney. We detox through the skin without having to do much at all, though exercising until we sweat and saunas help this process along. Our lungs help us to detoxify when we breathe, and exercising and sexing will increase the rate of breathing. The kidneys do the job of shuttling waste out through our urine. We can't, of course, forget the bowels, also known as the large intestine, where we collect waste matter to eliminate via a good poop. If our "doors" of elimination – the skin, lungs, kidney, and bowels – are closed off, things start to show up in other ways. We get breakouts on our skin and our eliminations most definitely don't smell like roses. Combine the toxins we're taking in with the toxins we're rubbing on, and the result is a big old mess that makes us want to layer more pretty-making toxic products on our skin.

What did you use this morning as you were getting ready? Yes. This is totally a trick question. But think about it. I imagine it's safe to assume toothpaste was involved and maybe a mouthwash. I am going to guess that you also washed your hands and maybe your body with soap, perhaps your hair too.

You may have used a shaving cream, a couple skin care products, some hair products, likely a bit of makeup, and then a spritz of your fave fragrance. Am I close?

According to the Environmental Working Group's Skin Deep Cosmetic Database, which rates the safety of brand-name products based on their ingredients, consumers use an average of ten personal-care products per day. Within those products, there are an estimated 126 ingredients. Currently, the government doesn't require health studies or pre-market testing for these products. Furthermore, in 2007 an Environmental Working Group analysis found that over the span of thirty years, the industry panel has reviewed the safety of just 11 percent of the 10,500 ingredients found in personal care products.[1] Yowza!

How many of those products would you eat? I'm serious. Would you take that cocktail of ten products you applied to your body and instead throw it in your blender, power her on up with some ice, and suck 'er down? Probably not, right?

I know what you're thinking. I thought it, too. If this stuff were so toxic and icky for us, there is no way we'd actually be allowed to use it. Part of the catch is that often these ingredients are tested in isolation. Meaning they test what one ingredient will do to us and it may seem totally safe. What happens when we combine eye shadow with eyeliner, mascara, makeup remover, and eye cream? One margarita likely won't hurt you, but one margarita combined with two shots of vodka, a banana daiquiri, some Grand Marnier, and a couple slices of pizza won't end well. Sometimes, when it comes to this stuff, we have to think about the sum of all the parts involved. This doesn't mean you have to whip out your patchouli oil, though it may not be sounding that bad after all. There are of course happy, healthy, safe, and equally luxurious options.

What I want you to think about as we trudge through what is often a tough lesson for peeps to grasp, especially women who give a lot of care to how they look and smell (and trust me, I am with you here), is that we are afraid to shake up our personal-care routine for fear that our complexion will explode, our eyelashes will fall out, and we'll suddenly look 131-years-old in bright daylight. Have no fear, my bathing beauty, we're going to get into the goodness that can make you glow from the inside out and of course from the outside in.

EDIBLE BEAUTY

You just be patient right now! I'm not going to jump ahead and just dish out the products you are supposed to use so you can just do a switchety-swap and carry on. I will get to that, but first I have some important tips on how you can actually eat your way to sunshiny, sparkling beauty, one bite at a time. These are the ultimate foods for beauty and what's so cool about this whole edible beauty thing is that when we start cooking up our cosmetics in the kitchen, we come to realize that the very same things that make us glow from the inside out can also make us glow from the outside in.

Let's have a look at the foods that make us radiate like the sixteen-year-old refreshed version of ourselves. Our UnDiet world is all about loading up on the goodness, so here are the goodest of the good to make us glow. This might help you to understand why your microdermabrasion isn't doing what the ad says when you follow it up with a coffee, two creams, and sugar.

Nutrients for the Morning-After Glow All Day

There are a few key goodies you want to look for when choosing foods that will nourish your skin. Here are my faves.

❊ **Fluids:** Fluids are the queen of the castle, as they help flush the waste and moisturize from the inside out. Remember, coffee is a diuretic, and it's going to make you pee like a racehorse while flushing vital nutrients and fluid, giving your skin the texture of a dried apricot. And p.s.: that second martini isn't doing you any more favors than the first.

Get Yours: Water, herbal tea, and green juice are at the top of the charts.

❊ **Essential Fatty Acids:** Omega-3s are the fatty acids we need for our skin to help bring down any inflammation and keep us nourished, smooth, and silky. In case you're wondering, ladies, omega-3s are also vital for creating a little natural lubrication down below. A self-lubricating woman is something sweet to strive for.

Get Yours: Walnuts, pecans, almonds, hazelnuts, Brazil nuts, flaxseeds, chia seeds, hemp seeds, and their oils are all fantabulous sources, as are organic eggs (with the yolk, please) and cold-water fish such as salmon, sardines, haddock, halibut, and trout.

❋ **Antioxidants:** I will say this just once: antioxidants in a face cream are a big-bottomed waste if you're not high-dosing on the goodies with your meals, too. These sweet little gems found in loads of plant-based food (beyond wine and chocolate, thank you very much) are a great line of defense against cellular damage caused by free radicals. They help protect us from infection and can help to prevent degenerative diseases such as cancer and heart disease. If you're looking old and beaten on the outside, it's a good sign that the same is happening on the inside.

Get Yours: Antioxidant powerhouse foods include berries, Brazil nuts, brightly colored veggies, and spices such as cinnamon, clove, and oregano.

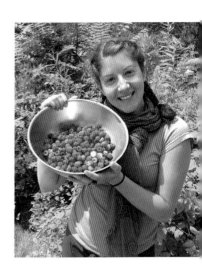

❋ **Vitamin A:** This is my fave vitamin for its awesome role in helping with the formation of new cells – mighty important for skin health. It helps keep our skin supple and is vital for the health of our eyes and hair. Watch out for bumps on the backs of your arms and thighs, a common sign of vitamin A deficiency.

Get Yours: Abundant in cold-water fish; organic eggs; dark orange veggies such as carrots, sweet potato, and butternut squash; and dark green veggies like broccoli, kale, and spinach.

❋ **Vitamin C:** This is one powerful antioxidant, which is why I love to include it in my diet, and also in my facemasks. Vitamin C is essential for the production of collagen, the elastic tissue in our skin. A decline in collagen is partly why we get all wrinkly as we age. Wanna know what kicks our vitamin C levels to the curb? Smoking, stress, and insufficient sleep.

Get Yours: Quit your vitamin C–depleting vices, get some sleep, and eat lots of red bell pepper, kale, parsley, citrus fruit, berries, and broccoli.

❋ **Vitamin E:** Another of my faves, vitamin E is a powerful defense against the damage of free radicals. As a fat-soluble nutrient, it's also part of the equation to help our skin retain moisture. Without enough vitamin E, we get premature wrinkling, paleness, acne, and easy bruising. Hot stuff!

Get Yours: Stock up on your nuts and seeds, whole grains, avocados, and sweet potatoes, and you'll be good to go.

❀ **Iron:** To put it simply, iron is a mineral that helps us have healthy, bright red blood. That healthy blood is what gives our skin a natural glow and helps keep the dark circles away from under our eyes.

Get Yours: High concentrations often come from animal foods, but I love to get me some iron-rich plant sources like pumpkin seeds, sea vegetables, leafy greens, lentils, and beans.

❀ **Selenium:** Selenium is awesometown in helping to protect our skin inside and out from free radical damage and dryness. It is necessary in the production of glutathione, a super-powered antioxidant, which neutralizes the free radicals in the body that can lead to the deterioration of collagen and elastin in the skin. It enhances the loveliness of our hair and nails.

Get Yours: Shake out that mane after you eat up your whole grains, organic eggs, beans, organic mushrooms, and Brazil nuts.

❀ **Zinc:** Bring on the zinc! It helps us manufacture collagen and it speeds up healing. A deficiency produces stretch marks, a dull complexion, dandruff, icky blemishes, and white spots on fingernails. Yep; that's what those white spots could mean. And let the men in your life know this handy rhyme: no zinc, no dink. The guys need zinc to play with us in the boudoir.

Get Yours: Are the foods looking familiar to you yet? Load up on the whole grains, free-run organic eggs, and nuts.

Now that you're on board with the role your salads, green juices, and nuts and seeds snacks are playing in your beauty routine, we are ready to get into the body-care-product cleanse.

WHAT'S THE BIG DEAL? IT'S JUST MOISTURIZER

The big deal is that toxins love to hang out in our fat. Sad but true. When we rub moisturizer on to our skin, we are *rubbing it in*, right? We want it to be absorbed and leave our skin feeling moisturized and smelling yummy. What we've just rubbed in, though, doesn't just stay on the surface of our skin, it soaks right on in, and everything in that cream has now entered our bloodstream and will begin to circulate. These chemicals might even be considered scarier than the ones we eat because they are actually bypassing the digestive system. Substances that absorb transdermally (through the skin), sublingually (under the tongue), or get inhaled (think beyond *those* kinds of inhaled substances to the everyday inhalants like the chlorine and fluoride in your shower water that is inhaled as a vapor) are bypassing the detox powerhouse that is the digestive system and liver, and going straight into circulation. This allows the toxins speedy access to the fat cells of our body (including the brain, which is mostly made up of fat). When the toxins overpower or bypass the body's many detox organs and processes, they begin to build up, weaken our natural defenses, alter DNA, and then, my home girls, things like cellulite, saggy aged skin, and even cancers start their parties.

Every single thing we put on our skin ends up in our body. If there are chemicals in a product we wouldn't eat, then why are we using them? Using chemical-laden products actually works to do the very opposite of what we want them to. We use them to look younger, but they are actually accelerating our journey toward looking like vintage leather luggage that's taken a few too many trips down the baggage carousel. Just like the edible poisons we've talked about, the cosmetic chemicals move on in, circulate, cause

DO YOU KNOW WHAT CELLULITE IS? It's ripples and dimples in the skin caused by **toxic build up** in the fat cells that have become stagnant. I am all about the self-love but learning to love a **cottage-cheese dimple bum** is a pretty challenging endeavor. **Massage** and dry-skin brushing regularly, in addition to lowering your intake and increasing your flushing out of toxins with loads of **water** and veggie juices, are the best strategies to **prevent** and diminish the old dimple-tushie.

free-radical damage and lo and behold, we age quicker, not to mention increase our risk of toxin-linked conditions such as autoimmune conditions and cancer.

There are now more than 75,000 known chemicals in our environment, most of which we can do very little about.[2] If we live in a city, spend any amount of time in traffic, go to public places, ride in airplanes, or hug friends who wear perfume, we're going to be exposed. It seems silly, then, not to do a little bit to reduce the load we inflict on ourselves. If we reduce our load of chemicals that we intake through our beauty regime designed to make us look younger, we actually will look younger. Bring on the patchouli! (Kidding. I promise. Just kidding.)

This Is Why You Need to Care about Beauty Care

THE BIG C: According to Dr. Samuel Epstein, chairman of the Cancer Prevention Coalition, cosmetics and personal-care products are perhaps the single most important, though mostly ignored, group of products that we can look out for to help prevent cancer, in our developed world.[3] I concur.

✽ **The Chemical Cocktail:** Even though a specific ingredient might not be in itself a proven carcinogen, it could very well be what is called a "hidden" carcinogen, meaning that under certain conditions, it can have carcinogenic properties, such as when it is combined with other substances in a product.

✽ **We Use Deodorant Every Day, Right?** Once in a while is no trouble at all, but think of all the things we use on a daily basis. Shmikees! The concern here is that daily exposure to toxic ingredients over a lifetime, many of which are left on the skin, have a cumulative effect – and not a good one.

✽ **Skin Absorbs. It's Just What It Does.** Our skin is like a sponge; we put the product on, the skin soaks it up. Think about your winter hand cream and lip-balm habit. How many times a day are you applying lip balm and hand cream? Any chemicals contained within those products keep soaking in as we keep reapplying. How many chemicals come along for the ride each time?

✽ **Wetting Agents Are What?** These are chemicals also known as surfactants that help reduce the surface tension of water. This essentially means they make stuff more absorbable. When they're added to a skincare product, they help it to rub in smoothly, often a selling feature when we're told an oil-based product has no oily residue. Wetting agents are chemicals that help creams absorb better. This is a problem because we don't want that stuff having an easier time getting in.

✽ **A Bypass of Our Enzyme Guards:** Carcinogens in personal-care products potentially pose greater cancer risks than foods that have carcinogenic pesticides and additives, because they bypass the digestive process. This means they also bypass the detox processes carried out by the liver and go straight into circulation, as I've mentioned.

Watch Out for These Bad Boys

Just as you have learned to read food labels and know what to watch out for, it's time to look out for cosmetic and personal-care product labels. "Natural" and "organic" don't mean a whole lot when it comes to packaged and processed foods, and the same can be said here. Let the ingredient labels tell the story. Here are some key ingredients you'll want to keep a watchful eye on.

COSMETIC ADDITIVE	FUNCTION	WHERE YOU'LL FIND IT	HEALTH RISK*
Alcohol (also called ethanol or ethyl alcohol)	Acts as a solvent, anti-foaming agent, and disinfectant; reduces viscosity (making substances less thick).	Mouthwash, astringents, toners, cleansers, and some toothpastes	Strips away skin's protecting oils, which can lead to more breakouts. In mouthwashes, it has been linked to mouth and throat cancers.
Aluminum	Reduces flow of sweat from the skin.	Antiperspirants and some cosmetics	Suspected link with central nervous system dysfunctions (such as Alzheimer's disease).
Coal tar dye	Used as a coloring agent and often an ingredient found in D&C Blue #1, Green #3, Yellow #5, Yellow #6, Red #33.	Dandruff shampoos, bubble bath, toothpastes, and hair dyes	A known human carcinogen and linked to severe allergic reactions, asthma attacks, headaches, nausea, fatigue, nervousness, lack of concentration, increased risk of non-Hodgkin's lymphoma, multiple myeloma, and Hodgkin's disease.

Diethanolamine (DEA), triethanolamine (TEA)	Solvent, emulsifier, and wetting agent.	Shampoos, conditioners, lotions, shaving gels, bubble bath, and skin cream	Known human carcinogen.
Fluoride (sodium fluoride)	An environmental pollutant that can contain lead, mercury, cadmium, arsenic, and radionuclides.	Toothpaste, whitening agents, and mouthwash	This heavy metal accumulates in the body and can inhibit thyroid function, contribute to bone disease, and is a known carcinogen.
Formaldehyde	Used as a preservative, fixative, and disinfectant.	Shampoo, nail care, baby products, deodorants, toothpaste, hairspray, and cosmetics	It is a suspected carcinogen and neurotoxin.
Fragrances (synthetic)	Synthetic fragrances are made up of hundreds of chemicals.	The majority of personal-care products: body washes, soaps, moisturizers, perfumes, shampoos, conditioners, etc.	Some, such as methylene chloride, are carcinogenic; others are linked to allergies, dermatitis, and respiratory and reproductive problems.
Mineral oil	A byproduct of the petroleum industry and makes skin feel soft and smooth.	Liquid foundations, blush, skin creams, and baby oil.	Inhibits the natural production of oils and so increases dehydration, clogs pores, locks in toxins and waste. Also linked to allergies and cancer.
Phthalates	A plastic softener. There are dozens of phthalates out there. Not always found on label of ingredients.	Hair spray, deodorant, nail polish, hair gel, mousse, hand lotion, body lotion, and perfume, as well as children's toys and PVC plastic	Shown to damage the liver, kidneys, lungs, and reproductive system, especially in developing testes.
Propylene glycol	Prevents things from drying out.	Deodorants, shampoos, conditioners, lotions, and shaving gels	Implicated in contact dermatitis, kidney damage, and liver abnormalities. Can damage cell membranes, causing rashes, dry skin, and surface damage.

Sodium lauryl sulfate (SLS)	A detergent derived from coconut oil (can be called "natural" or even "organic") and makes things foamy.	Toothpaste, shampoo, dish soap, liquid hand soap, and bubble bath	Builds up in the heart, liver, lungs, and brain from skin contact; may cause damage to these organs. Corrodes hair follicles and impairs ability to grow hair, may cause hair to fall out.
Talc	Prevents caking, adds bulk, absorbs moisture, and protects skin.	Baby powders, feminine powders, blush, lubricant on condoms	Proven carcinogen when inhaled, used topically, or in genital areas.

*Source: Environmental Working Group's Skin Deep Data base, http://www.ewg.org/skindeep.

KEY STEPS IN UNDIETING THE BEAUTY ROUTINE

Don't go into panic mode. You know I have your back and we're going to take baby steps together to clean up our beauty act. Just as wiping your cupboards clear of years of eating habits in one fell swoop would be a massive waste of goods and expense, same goes for the cosmetic cabinet. We're going to break down the clean up into five easy steps.

❋ **Assess the Poison:** What are the goods you believe you must, must, must have and cannot even begin to contemplate a substitution for? What are the goods you use because you think you are supposed to have them but don't really notice any difference (eye cream comes to mind)? What are the goods you use every day? What are the products you use once in a while?

❋ **Replace the Everyday:** Things you use every single day — deodorant, toothpaste, hand soap, moisturizer, and fragrance — replace as soon as possible with a lean and clean option.

❋ **Less Is More:** Try using a smaller quantity of everything that you are using now. This is an easier transition for some than just getting rid of everything. There is no need to soap up your face day and night, and does hair really need a shampoo every day? We live in a pretty clean place and unless you're

Germaphobe? Anyone else a little creeped by the amount of hand sanitizer being doled out? Scientists at the University of Ireland found that using chemical disinfectants could actually lead to the growth of superbugs that become resistant to both the cleansers and antibiotics.[4] A super option is to work with the power of nature and try some potent antimicrobial essential oils such as tea tree, clove, cinnamon, or eucalyptus.

on a farm shoveling compost or it's the middle of a heat wave, you only need to soap up the pits and the bits (see below left).

❄ **Special Occasion Items:** Make some of your products that you don't want to replace, such as nail polish, perfume, and hair dye, your very special occasion items, though be well aware there are amazing less-toxic options available. A manicure is not essential (and can add a massive toxic load) and I'll bet you love your own perfume more than anyone else does. You know that person who works near you who wears that horrible fragrance and way too much of it? Chances are good that someone else thinks the same about yours. Fragrance is the new second-hand smoke. There, I said it.

❄ **Transition to Better Choices:** When you have to replace products, make smarter choices. Check out the Environmental Working Group's online Cosmetic Database. With more than 69,000 products on there, look up some brands and find the low-chemical, clean-loving options.

ARE WE SOAPING OFF OUR VITAMIN D?

We can get vitamin D from the sun, right? This is one of the many reasons we're told to hit the sunshine without protection for about ten minutes a day. We're missing an important link, though. Vitamin D3 is an oil-soluble steroid hormone that is formed when your skin is exposed to ultraviolet B (UVB) from the sun. It is formed on the surface of your skin and doesn't absorb straight away. It actually takes up to **forty-eight hours** before we are able to absorb the majority of the vitamin D generated by the sun into our skin.[5] After a hot day, when we shower off and scrub from head to toe with soap, we're washing that vitamin D right down the drain. To optimize your vitamin D levels, try and **delay washing** the whole entire body with soap for about two full days after sun exposure. Please don't stop bathing! But perhaps you want to limit your soap use to just the pits and bits.

EAT IT UP AND SLATHER IT ON

What's really cool about all of the edible beauty products I am about to introduce to you is that they make the most amazing beauty routine, whether we're prettying on up by eating the goods or literally smearing them up, down, and all around our beautiful faces and deliciously hot bodies.

The best part, of course, about UnDieting our beauty routine is that, almost instantly and without much effort, we have dramatically lightened the load of questionable chemicals we are taking in, as well as the garbage we're making. Remember that rule about real food and avoiding stuff that has to pay a visit to the chemistry lab before it lands on our table? We should apply that to the goods that go on our skin. Call me crazy (if you haven't yet), but I don't really want to put something on my face that had to be tested to ensure it won't burn a hole through my skin or cause my hair to fall out of my head. Try these instead.

Keep It Lubed: Keep three jars of coconut oil handy: one for the kitchen for cooking, one in the bathroom for all your beauty needs, and one in the bedroom for a little bow-chica-bow-bow slip-sliding action.

FOOD FOR BEAUTY	FUNCTION	FAVE USES
Aloe	Helps soothe burns and pain, and promotes accelerated wound healing. Also antibacterial and antimicrobial.	Apply topically to any burns, whether from the sun or the stove. Also great for cuts as an antibacterial.
Apple cider vinegar	Highly alkalinizing, astringent, and rich in minerals; makes it ideal for balancing pH on skin.	Dilute 1:10 with water for an astringent/toner, hair rinse, and scalp tonic.
Avocado	All of those good fats in the avocado make them ideal for moisturizing and nourishing the skin.	Apply to skin of the face for a deep moisturizing mask, or to hair to promote growth.
Baking soda (aluminum-free)	Rich with loads of components that help to neutralize pH and also acts as a mild abrasive substance.	Add a pinch to your toothbrush for gentle polishing or to a little to water to create a mild exfoliating face scrub.
Buffered vitamin C powder	Potent antioxidant; great for preserving smooth, youthful skin and promoting wound healing·	Mix into your homemade face mask for extra rejuvenating benefit.
Cucumber	Nourishing, hydrating, and cooling properties make it ideal for problem skin areas.	Apply thin cool slices to the eyes to bring down puffiness, reduce dark circle inflammation, and irritation from rashes.
Coconut oil (cold-pressed)	Antimicrobial, antiviral, antifungal, and anti-bacterial, this is an ideal oil to use all over the body and on the hair.	Use as a daily moisturizer, gentle eye makeup remover, or deep pre-shampoo conditioning treatment.

Green tea	Power punch of antioxidants.	Use green tea as a steam, the leaves as an exfoliant, or allow the tea to cool for an effective breath freshening mouthwash.
Lavender essential oil	Antimicrobial, antiviral, antifungal, and anti-bacterial properties makes this ideal for topical infection, soothing, and to promote healing.	Add to coconut oil for overall beauty, a couple drops in the pits for deodorant, or a dab under the nose to reduce stress and bring forth a beautiful glowing smile.
Lemon	Rich in antioxidants, alkalinizing, and disinfecting.	Rub lemon on elbows, knees, and cracked heels to speed healing, or use on hands to get rid of cooking odors. Mix with water for an extra-shine hair rinse.
Oats	Anti-irritant and anti-inflammatory properties, as well as moisturizing and soothing.	Use as a facial and/body exfoliant. Mix with raw honey to make a nourishing face mask.
Raw cocoa	Extra rich in antioxidants and a natural source of magnesium – perfect combo for anti-aging and defense against environmental elements.	Mix into a mask with avocado or make a paste with water for a face or body mask.
Raw honey	Antimicrobial, antiviral, antifungal, and anti-bacterial, rich in enzymes, and promotes healing.	Use topically for burns, add to avocado and cocoa for a face mask, mix with sea salt or oats for a scrub.
Sea salt	Rich in minerals and very alkalinizing.	Use as mouth rinse to alkalize the mouth as defense against bacteria and plaque. Add to honey or oats for face or body scrub.

LET COSMETICS BE YOUR MEDICINE: ESSENTIAL OILS FOR BEAUTY CARE BY NADINE ARTEMIS

Essential oils, the aromatic molecules of plant life, are a botanical blessing for beautifying the whole being.

❋ **Rose Otto:** A single drop of rose otto (also called attar of roses), the fairest of all botanical oils, requires sixty fragrant roses to lend out their aromatic juices. Since ancient days, humans have relied on rose otto to heal our critical connective tissues, repairing both broken hearts and wrinkled skin. Beautifying for all skin types, this essential oil improves the skin's elasticity and resiliency, and speeds up skin repair.

❈ **Sea Buckthorn Berry:** Bursting with nutrition, one drop of sea buckthorn berry extract captures more than 190 skin-blessing substances! Rich in essential fatty acids (EFAs), this bright orange berry is also full of antioxidants, carotenoids, and phytosterols. Absorbing deeply into the skin, sea buckthorn solves the root cause of skin irritating imbalances.

❈ Lavender: Sweetly soothing lavender is one of the gentlest, yet most healing, essential oils for skin care. Therapeutic and restorative, its anti-inflammatory and regenerative properties heal burns, prevent scarring, and even out worried skin – and a worried mood.

❈ Frankincense: Frankincense delivers clarity in all things, including the skin. Traditionally used to treat scar tissue and skin ulcers, this essntial oil also replenishes dry and prematurely aging skin, improving its resiliency and texture. Frankincense soothes the mind and the nerves.

❈ **Immortelle:** Immortelle revivifies every filament of your being. This highly praised healer promotes cell rejuvenation while reducing inflammation and redness. It is a beautiful treatment for bruises, scars, and blemishes.

Innovative aromacologist Nadine Artemis is the creator of Living Libations. Her exquisite beauty formulas, medicinal blends, and potent dental serums have received rave reviews and she is an acclaimed presenter on natural wellness and renegade beauty.

YOU PUT FOOD ON YOUR COUNTERS, RIGHT?

I'm not gonna lie. I miss the smell of lemon-fresh chemical cleaner. When I was in university, cleaning days were like days off from school and I would scrub my apartment with the best of the worst chemical cleaners because I liked that "clean" smell. Little did I know that the very best "clean" smell is actually no smell at all, and that nauseatingly weird smell is actually a cocktail of chemical crappola.

If we're going to start cleaning up what goes on our body, we also have to think about the stuff that touches our skin and what we inhale while cleaning. If you put food on your counters and dishes, have small children, have big children, have pets, or live in a home, then clean it right! We're taking this to the next level and UnDieting our full toxic load.

This is where you really get to save some moolah too, so you can spend extra on your organic veggies for your juicing needs.

Basic Home Cleaning Ingredients

* **Baking Soda:** Cleans, deodorizes, softens water, and scours.
* **Natural Soap or Detergent:** This can come as unscented in liquid form, flakes, powders, or bars. In this form it is biodegradable and will cleanse just about anything.
* **Lemon:** As one of the strongest food acids, fresh lemon juice is awesomely effective in disinfecting household bacteria.
* **Borax:** Yep, just like they used in the Old Country. This classic cleaning ingredient deodorizes, disinfects, softens water, and cleans painted walls and floors for those times you explode smoothies across your kitchen. Really, as if I'm the only one.
* **White Vinegar:** Mix with water as a produce cleaner, and also great to clean grease, remove mildew, deodorize, and help keep your poached eggs together. Well, it does.
* **Tea Tree Oil:** One of the strongest natural antiseptics – makes it great in a surface cleaner (add it to mop water), and a fantastic addition to any all-purpose cleaner.

Best Home-Cleaning Concoctions

❉ All-Purpose Cleaner: Mix ½ cup (125 mL) vinegar and ¼ cup (50 mL) baking soda (or 2 tsp/10 mL borax) into 6 cups (1.5 L) of water. Use to remove water-deposit stains from shower-stall panels, bathroom chrome fixtures, windows, bathroom mirrors, etc.

❉ Disinfectant: Mix 2 tsp (10 mL) borax, ¼ cup (50 mL) vinegar, and 3 cups (750 mL) hot water. For stronger cleaning power add ¼ tsp (1 mL) liquid soap and a couple drops of tea tree oil. Wipe surfaces with dampened cloth.

❉ Drain Cleaner: For a basic drain cleaning, mix ½ cup (125 mL) salt in 1 gallon (4 L) of water, heat (not boil! Plastic pipes can melt) the mix and pour down the drain. For a more powerful cleaning, pour ½ cup (125 mL) baking soda down the drain followed by a ½ cup (125 mL) vinegar. The resulting chemical reaction can break fatty acids down, allowing the clog to wash down the drain. After 15 minutes, pour in hot water to clear residue.

❉ Deodorizer: Place partially filled saucers of vinegar around the room or simmer a pot of warm water containing a few drops of your favorite essential oil.

❉ Natural Toilet Bowl Cleaner: Sprinkle baking soda into the bowl, then drizzle with vinegar and scrub down with a toilet brush. This task is helped out by having cute cleaning gloves. Be warned, it's best not to mix the combo with store-bought toilet cleaners for fear of hazardous fumes.

❉ Glass Cleaner: I learned this one from my Mozambican room-mate when I was living in Australia (a story for another book). Mix equal amounts of water and vinegar in a spray bottle. Spritz away and then wipe the glass or mirror with newspaper.

Safety First! Do not attempt the natural cleaning solutions after using commercial options, as dangerous fumes or unpredictable, adverse chemical reactions can occur.

Common chemicals found in everyday cosmetics and cleaning products are dousing us in poison. It's easy to get hooked on the stuff. Cutting out toxic nail polish will have no negative effects on your quality of life, nor will switching from a toxic cleaning spray to one that doesn't bear a skull and crossbones. The effect on your radiant complexion can be massive in a good way. You can still wear makeup, style your hair, and look gorge-alicious. You're just going to be a little smarter about it. Understood?

Imagine how your liver, skin, and other detox organs would sing if they didn't have to be choking on the chemicals we throw at them daily. If UnDiet is about simplifying our living for vibrant health, then this really is the next logical place to take our transitions. We worry about the water we drink and the quality of our food, but then we go and junk ourselves up with all these scary chemicals. There is simply no need. Sometimes we're better off just rocking it like it's 1856, eating clean food, and seeing where our creativity takes us in working out whole and healthy ways to luxuriate in simple decadence.

UNDIET LIVING

UnDiet for Abundance Mantra

If it doesn't belong inside, it's not being smeared on the outside.

Make Love in the Kitchen

Remove the chemical factory from our body and home.

* No indulging in expensive beauty-care treatments and products. Time to eat your way beautiful.
* Ditch the toxic cleaning products. Finish what you have and do better next time.
* No need to be a product hoarder. Reduce the amount of cosmetic and personal-care products used on a daily basis.
* Farewell to the daily chemical bath you've been taking in all those processed cosmetic products.

TRANSITIONAL TIPS AND TRICKS TO MAKE IT HAPPEN

* **Go without.**
  Can you shed the make-up? Choose three days out of the week that you limit your makeup to a little lip gloss.
* **Cut down on what you use.**
  Choose 50 percent of your daily products that you will continue using as regular products. Reserve the rest as special occasion goodies.
* **Replace.**
  Do your research and replace the goods that you are using on a daily basis with safer options. Either make the replacements yourself or choose non-toxic lotions and potions.
* **Mix your own.**
  Spend an hour mixing up your new home cleaning products. Please, please, please do the right thing and use up or get rid of your old stuff responsibly. (Dumping them down the drain is not responsible.)
* **Take it to the bank.**
  Determine what you spend on average, each year, on manicures, hair dyes, cosmetics, and personal-care products. Now that you've cut down, see what you'll save each week and create a fund. Spend that on other forms of beauty care like massages, acupuncture, or a holiday.

DRIED
LEMON BALM

DRIED
CALENDULA

DRIED
SAGE

DRIED
CHAMOMILE

DRIED
LAVENDER

DRIED
LEMON PEEL

DRIED
ROSEMARY

APPLE CIDER
VINEGAR

Apple Cider Astringent or Toner (page 209)

Apple Cider Astringent or Toner

½ cup	dried lemon balm	125 mL
⅓ cup	dried chamomile	75 mL
¼ cup	dried calendula	50 mL
¼ cup	dried lavender	50 mL
1 tbsp	dried lemon peel	15 mL
1 tbsp	dried part rosemary	15 mL
1 tbsp	dried part sage	15 mL
	Apple cider vinegar to cover	

DIRECTIONS

- Place the herbs in a wide-mouth jar. Add enough vinegar so that it rises 2 or 3 inches (8 or 10 cm) above the mixture.
- Cover jar tightly and shake the mixture. Add more vinegar if needed to ensure the herbs are completely covered.
- Every day for 2 weeks, shake the mixture to ensure the herbs are always fully covered. After 2 weeks, strain out the herbs using a nut sack or sieve.
- Mix 1 tbsp (15 mL) of vinegar mixture with ¾ cup (175 mL) water. This is your toner!
- Label and store remaining vinegar for later use. This does not need to be refrigerated and will keep indefinitely.

Get Fancy: Dilute this recipe with water, witch hazel, or rose water for a fancy-pants astringent, toner, or hair rinse. Store it in a glass spray bottle, and you have the perfect after-shower body spray.

The One-to-Two Rule: You can always replace dried herbs in recipes with fresh by doubling the amount. For example: 1 tbsp of dried lemon peel is equivalent to 2 tbsp of fresh.

Pretty Me Latte

¼ cup	raw cocoa powder	50 mL
2 tbsp	coconut oil	30 mL
2 tbsp	hemp seeds	30 mL
½	avocado	½
1 tsp	buffered vitamin C powder (optional)	5 mL
3 cups	warm water	750 mL
	pinch of sea salt	
	raw honey to taste	

DIRECTIONS

- Blend all the ingredients in your high-speed blender until smooth.
- Drink up.

Edible Body Butter

¼ cup	cocoa butter	50 mL
1 tbsp	grated beeswax	15 mL
2 tbsp	baking powder	30 mL
1 tbsp	extra virgin olive oil	15 mL
10 drops	essential oil of choice	10 drops

DIRECTIONS

- In a double boiler (one medium pot filled with water, with a smaller pot floating inside), melt together cocoa butter, beeswax, coconut oil, and extra virgin olive oil.
- Stir in essential oil and quickly pour into storage container, like a 4 oz glass jar.
- Store in cupboard; to harden quicker, store in fridge. Depending on the season, this blend will be firm or more liquid. The more beeswax used, the more solid it will be.

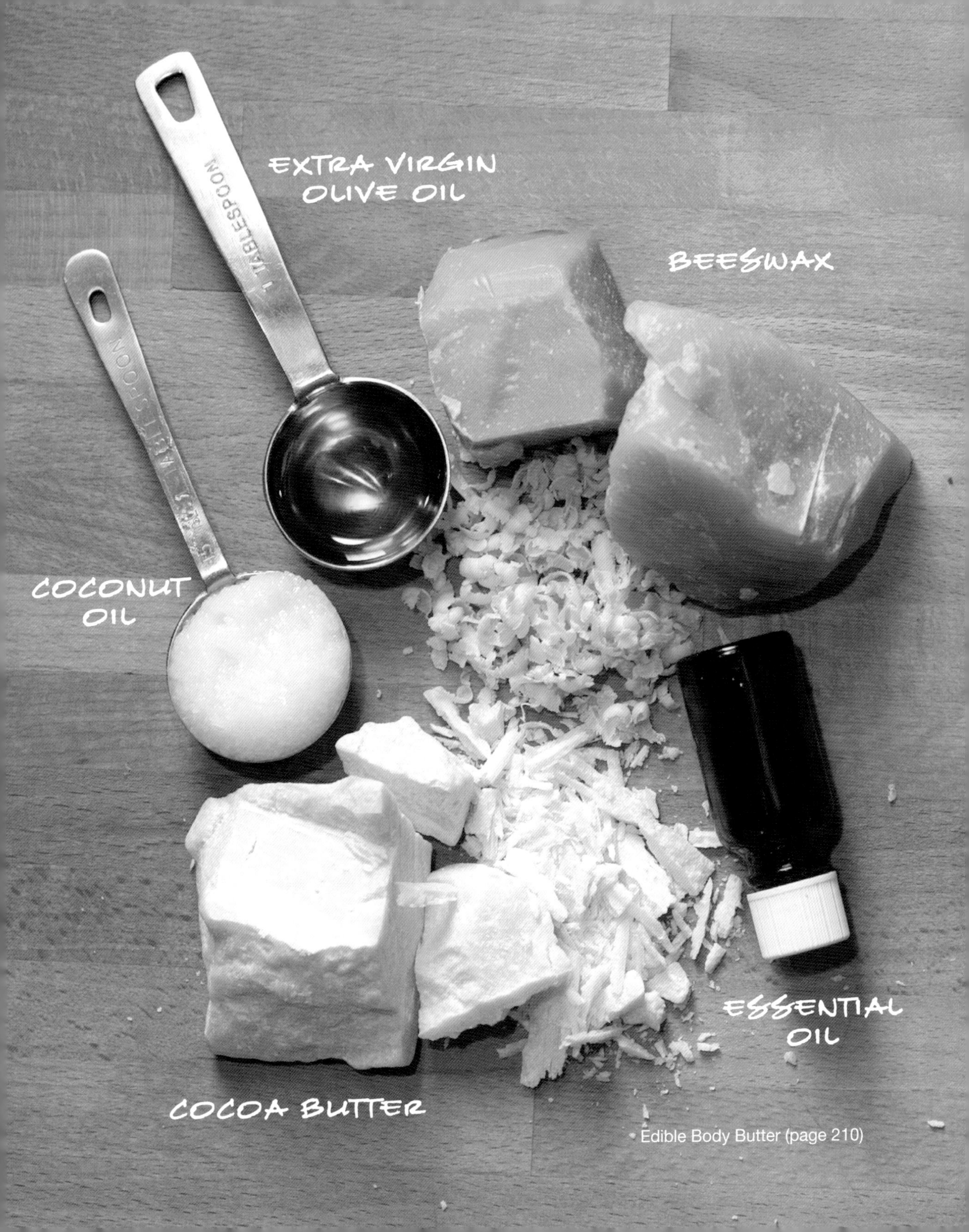

EXTRA VIRGIN
OLIVE OIL

BEESWAX

1 TABLESPOON

COCONUT
OIL

COCOA BUTTER

ESSENTIAL
OIL

Edible Body Butter (page 210)

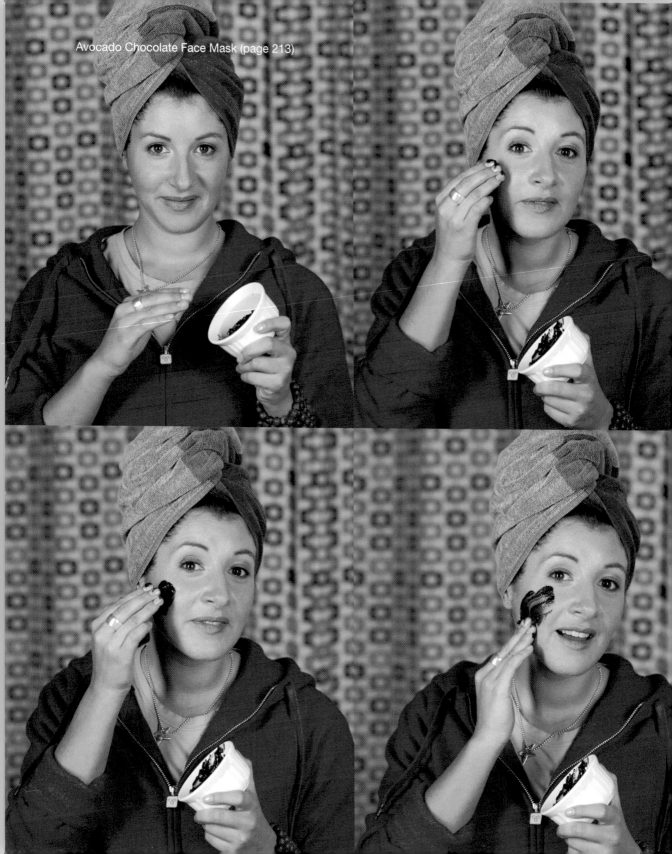
Avocado Chocolate Face Mask (page 213)

Avocado Chocolate Face Mask (or Cupcake Frosting)

¼ cup	raw honey	50 mL
¼ cup	raw cocoa powder	50 mL
½	avocado	½
1 tbsp	coconut oil	15 mL
2 tsp	buffered vitamin C powder (optional)	10 mL
1 tbsp	fresh aloe (optional)	15 mL
2 drops	lavender essential oil (optional)	2 drops

DIRECTIONS

- Place all ingredients into food processor and blend until smooth, or use large mixing bowl and a fork and mash until smooth.
- Gently rinse face with warm water and apply mask to the face. Leave on for 10–15 minutes.
- Rinse with warm water and pat dry.

All-Natural Breath Rinse

2 cups	water	500 mL
2 tsp	vodka (optional)	10 mL
1 tbsp	sea salt	15 mL
4	drops peppermint essential oil	4
2	drops clove essential oil (optional)	2
1	drop lemon essential oil (optional)	1

DIRECTIONS

- Mix all ingredients together in jar.
- Shake bottle well before pouring out serving.
- Rinse mouth thoroughly, swishing water around teeth, and spit.
- Repeat as necessary.

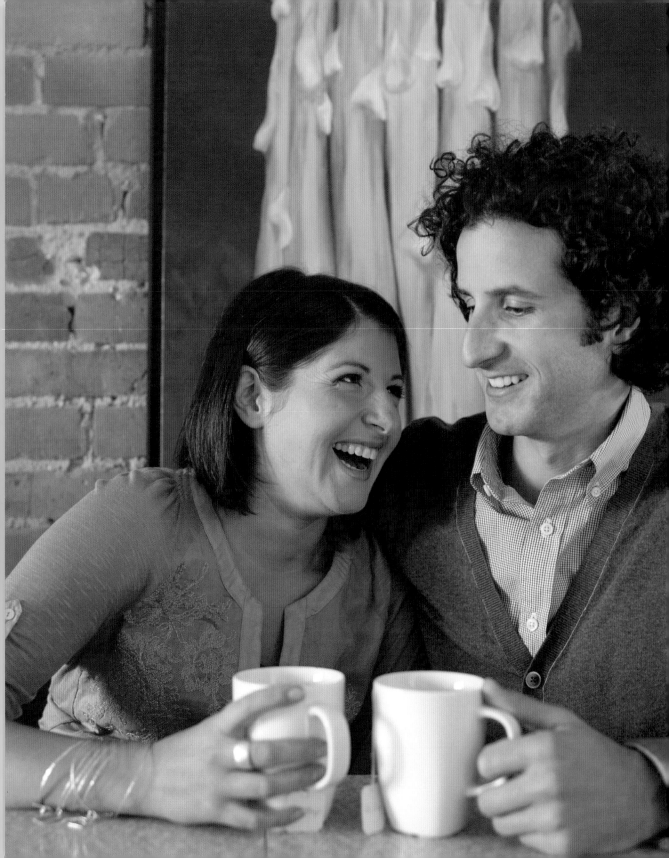

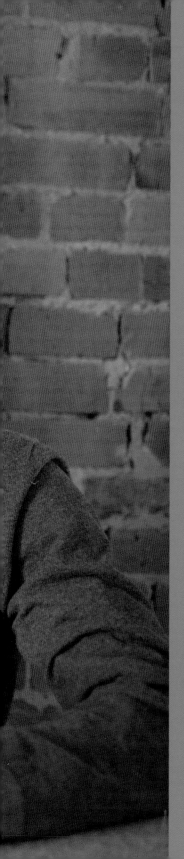

CHAPTER 10

Love What You Do and Do It with Love

When it comes to natural health and natural healing, there is simply no single solution and no overnight miracle. It all takes time, commitment, and love. UnDieting is a commitment to a whole lot of love for yourself. The act of consuming things, thinking things, doing things, and being around people who drag us down is the greatest act of disrespect we can subject ourselves to. The healthier we become in both our body and mind, the more love we want to dress up in. We begin to feel more deserving of it as we start feeling more alive and more vibrant. The daily struggles of getting enough sleep, drinking enough water, and passing on the cupcakes become the non-negotiable easy-breezy parts of our lives. We do the right things for ourselves because these small choices and habits enhance our life, make us feel amazing, and contribute to the prosperity in every other aspect of our life. And we deserve it a thousand and five times over.

"Feeling grateful or appreciative of someone or something in your life actually attracts more of the things that you appreciate and value into your life."
– Dr. Christiane Northrup

At this point, if you've been playing along with the game plan, you are likely feeling it. The tough stuff has passed, you've soaked up the information and you are glowing with abundant sasstastic energy. The ease that begins to rain down when we stop believing that achieving our goals has to be some kind of torturous struggle is truly remarkable. If we simply stop focusing on what we can't have and look at all the awesometown awesomeness that we can have, continuing to break the rules we've been taught, and living the life of our dreams becomes the easiest thing ever in the whole wide and wise world.

You know the phrases "in a perfect world" or "in an ideal world"? We use them all the time. Here's the thing, my little coconut: This is the only world we have. Yes, that storm cloud is going to come by once in a while and dump a load of disaster, crisis, upset, disappointment, pain, and struggle all over us right after we've put on our best new party dress, but is that any reason to never get dressed up? The poop of life is inevitable. You know what else is also inevitable? That the storm cloud will pass, the sun will shine, and you bet your bottom dollar that when the sun comes out tomorrow, I will be dressed to the nines and be ready to kick up my heels and party. Why set a limit to only ever seeing the glass as half empty or half full? Let's get that magenta fancy-pants smoothie glass overflowing with all that life serves up to us. The good with the bad, home-slizzle. The good with the bad.

In this final transitional phase of the UnDiet, now that our eating habits are renewed and revived, as are our low-impact ways and natural-beauty glow, it is time to get down to the last and most critical bits and pieces: the moving, shaking, sleeping, thinking, and being.

SHAKE THAT BOOTY

As eight-year-old girls, my best friend Macy and I would spend entire afternoons choreographing dance routines. Techno Tronic's "Pump up the Jam," Janet Jackson's "Revolution," Paula Abdul's "Straight Up," and Tiffany's "I Think We're Alone Now" were our tunes of choice. We'd get suited up in quasi-coordinated, too-cool-for-elementary-school, late-eighties acid-wash overalls and bust out the moves for whoever's parents were around to watch. We'd be tired, breathless, and smiling from top to bottom by the end of the shenanigans.

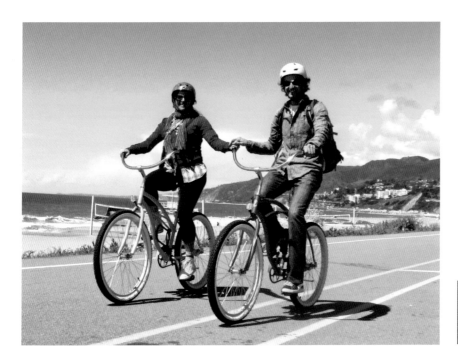

get the stories
behind the photos
http://bit.ly/UnDiet

That's what working out and getting our sweat on should be like as grown-ups.

Exercise should be fun. I'm not suggesting that going to the gym, lifting weights, running on a treadmill, or being pushed by a trainer isn't fun. If you love it and it works for you, awesome. Go, do it, love it, and reap the benefits.

I am guessing, however, that many peeps out there don't love the gym, but resign themselves to it as something that must be done. Did you know that there are other ways to exercise? Allow me to free you of your exercise burden. And, no, this is not an excuse to do nothing. It's actually quite the opposite. If you are going to get any benefit at all from working out, getting your heart rate up, building muscle, pumping up your metabolic rate, and getting that healthy glow on, you are going to have to either learn to love the workouts you currently do or fall in love with a whole new approach to achieving those benefits. It has to be within your means, make you feel awesome, get you the results you want, and most importantly, you must enjoy it to bits.

Make a choice and don't let your mind kick your ass instead of letting the workout kick it (and likely tighten it and lift it up off the backs of your legs too). Also know that a walk, or a gentle home practice of yoga may not give you the same benefits as a power run, but you know what? You'll still get more benefit physically than doing nothing at all, and chances are good that if you are feeling too physically tired to run, you're likely getting more benefit by being a little gentle on yourself. That can be the toughest part of all – being okay with ease sometimes.

The part for you to figure out is what type of exercise you love to do most and go and do it. It doesn't have to be about carving out two hours, three times a week for a high-intensity workout if you never end up making the time to do it. Perhaps what may work better for you is one hour a few times a week or perhaps even better might be twenty minutes every day. I am of the mindset that consistency trumps all else. If you can do it regularly with effort and a positive outlook and enjoy the process, it will be that much easier to maintain.

Balancing exercises do more than strengthen the physical body. Balancing poses in yoga can be some of the toughest, and are believed to help calm and strengthen the nervous system. Being calm when uncomfortable is a skill like any other and needs to be practiced in order to be strengthened. A great practice is learning to laugh when your balance is off and you have a bit of a stumble. Laughing when you stumble and fall – there is a practice worth taking off your mat and out into the world.

THE BOOTY-SHAKING OPTIONS ARE ENDLESS

Beyond going to the gym, there are a gazillion forms of exercise that you can take on. Often, you don't need to even leave your house if you have a computer nearby for guidance and motivation. You can do crazy intense sweaty yoga and the only equipment you need is a mat and a little rectangle of floor. You can tone the tummy and bring your sexy back with a hula hoop. I love the idea of a grown-up's jungle gym (also known as an indoor climbing wall); spin classes; trail hiking and biking; hot, ashtanga, hatha, or vinyasa yoga; belly dancing (which helps us learn to love the jiggle in the middle); or even just a long walk with some great music around your neighborhood. If you live in a bigger city, there are likely more out-of-the-box, fun-in-the-sun options to choose from. Mix it up.

❧ **Stamina:** This is often called aerobics or endurance training where you get that heart rate pumping and the sweat sweating.

❧ **Strength:** This is when resistance or weight-bearing activity comes into play. Strength training will keep us toned and taut and helps elevate our metabolic rate over a longer period of time. Strength training is what helps us burn up our flabbidy-flab.

❧ **Flexibility:** Slow, easy, stretching is going to help improve our range of motion, enable us to really get down when we boogie, and pick ourselves back up. It helps prevent injury when you attempt that back flip at your best friend's wedding or when you pick up a child.

❧ **Balance:** This is more than standing on one leg, though that helps. Good balance, as you may have worked out, helps prevent falling down, which may not seem too important to you right now, but one day it will, so you best start working on this (see page 218).

❧ **Core:** We need a strong core to maintain a healthy, strong lower back and good posture. A strong core is essentially the foundation for all the exercise we do and is vital to help prevent injury.

❧ **Warm Up and Cool Down:** Like any good roll in the hay with your lover, your workout needs the same kind of progression. I know, sometimes quickies are fun and when it comes to a workout, you just want to get it on and get 'er done. Slow down, Speedy. Warm yourself as you ease into it, hit your peak, and gently calm right on down.

❧ **Progress:** It may be a bit tough to track your progress in a private dance party for one, where you aim to successfully complete a "thread the needle," headstand or specific crunking move, but in general you want to keep pushing yourself just enough. Stagnation is lame, so keep switching things up and moving onwards and upward. Give your body a reason to change and adapt.

TIPS TO TRANSFORM THAT BOD
BY SAMMIE KENNEDY

Everybody is looking for the magic solution to achieving the fit and healthy body they desire. There is no "magic pill" or quick-fix solution to losing weight, toning your body, or just reaching a high level of athleticism. There are, however, a few secrets to the success of those ladies that actually reach their goals.

❀ **Own it!** Success comes with responsibility. Until you decide that you are indeed responsible for achieving your *own* results, even the small things can throw you off track. Once you have truly resolved and committed to changing your health through exercise, excuses have no room. You are responsible for your workouts; schedule them in and remain focused.

❀ **List it!** Exactly why do you want to lose weight? Do 40 pushups? Run a marathon? Listing out at least 25 reasons as to why you are committed to reaching your goal creates a compelling argument for why you should *not* fall off the wagon. Referring this list when you are feeling discouraged can help you refocus and recommit to your new healthy lifestyle.

❀ **Eat it!** No healthy body can survive on exercise alone. If you are seeking a truly healthy body that radiates fitness from the inside out, you can't neglect the inside part! Your toned muscles, smooth and tight skin, and healthy heart and lungs are not built solely from sprints and squats; they are built by the fuel and nutrients you put inside your body. No exercise regime will give you a body that glows with health without being paired with a nutrient-dense culinary lifestyle.

Sammie Kennedy is the creator and CEO of Booty Camp Fitness, Canada's largest boot camp program designed exclusively for women. She is also the CEO and creator of Femme Fitale, a women's mixed martial and kickboxing program.

SLEEP UNTIL YOU CAN'T SLEEP NO MORE

There is nothing I love more than watching people do the head mambo on public transit and airplanes. I am simultaneously enthralled, in awe, and entertained. Part of my fixation on this is because people just look funny with their head bouncing here and there as they fall in and out of sleep, but also because I am pretty sure I have never been tired enough to successfully accomplish the head mambo.

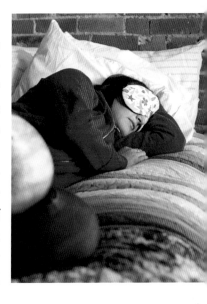

There are so many reasons to get a good night's sleep: it boosts our immune function, and improves our cognitive processes, our mood, and our metabolism. Sadly, when we get busy, sleep seems to be the first thing to go. Of all the things we can do for our health, this really should be at the top of our list and we don't do it nearly enough. What's so amazing about this little task for optimal health is that you don't actually have to do anything, just lie down and breathe. Even better – you get to do this naked if you want!

UnDiet Tips for Great Sleep

❀ **Eat Your Way to Sleepy.** No, this is not about eating until you are too tired to move, but about making the best food choices to help promote a restful state. Chlorophyll-rich foods, such as leafy green vegetables, raw or lightly steamed, are some of the best. Fruits such as mulberries and lemons help to calm the mind while whole grains boost serotonin levels, the feel-good chemical in our brain and gut. Say toodles to stimulants like alcohol, sugar, caffeine, and ciggies late in the day and into the night (or forever, always!).

❀ **Schedule Your Sleep.** Generally we need eight hours of sleep a night to maintain health. Going to bed and getting up at the same time every day will do wonders for your sleep cycle. Old patterns can be hard to break, as you well know by now, but if you can start getting up at the same time, resisting an afternoon nap, and going to sleep at the same time, you'll be amazed how quickly your body falls into the pattern.

❀ **Magic Happens in the Dark.** Keep your bedroom as dark and as quiet as possible. The littlest amount of ambient light from your alarm clock, from streetlamps, or even around the edge of your door can inhibit your ability to

Bedtime Alert! Setting an alarm to tell us when to wake up is common practice. What about setting an alarm to tell us when it is time to get prepped and ready for bed? Do it! Set an alarm as the signal to shut down the lights, turn off all electronics, have a cup of tea, or take a bath – something to transition you to bedtime. Plan to be in bed with the lights out one hour after the alarm sounds.

fall into a deep slumber. If black-out blinds are not an option or won't do the trick, a sleep mask can work wonders.

❋ **Create a Sanctuary.** Make your bedroom a place for calmness and cuddles. This means work or school materials have no place in your love den. Keep the pets (and children) out of your bed, as they have different sleep patterns and often move around in bed, causing us to wake during the night. Also, be sure to open a window a crack or turn the heat down. We sleep better in a cooler environment.

❋ **Let's Get It On!** Yes, I'm talking sexy sex. Get it on, in pairs, on your own, or whatever does the trick for you. Sex helps release tension, and gets the mind off the day to day. During orgasm, the chemical oxytocin is released, promoting sleep (though this is no excuse for him passing out immediately after). Do it and do it often!

Sleep rituals are handy dandy and your computer and television should never be a part of them. The bedroom should be reserved for sleeping and loving. I am also a big fan of foot and back massages, dimming the lights, and perhaps inhaling a little lavender. Warning: these may lead to the final point above.

TEN LITTLE BIG GAME CHANGERS

Sometimes it's simply the littlest habits that we take on that make the greatest impact on our health. Exercise and sleep are two of the biggest, but it can be these seemingly unimportant tasks or changes that add up to making the really big stuff not just possible, but easy. Presented in no particular order, these are the things we need to make time for every single day, no matter what.

1 **Dry Skin Brush:** Using a dry skin brush or even a dry loofah, start at your feet and brush, brush, brush your way up your legs, up your torso, from your hands, along your arms to your chest. The skin is the largest and most important elimination organ in the body and works really hard to get rid of all the toxic waste we accumulate. We eliminate approximately two pounds of waste material each day, mainly through our sweat glands. Super cool is that dry skin brushing can also be used as a preventative treatment for dry skin, as it stimulates ongoing skin renewal and is equally awesome for moving the lymph through our body to boost our immune system. Added bonus: it lends a gentle rub and tug to those fat cells we talked about earlier that store toxins and give us the old cottage-cheese dimple cellulite bum. Three months of daily dry skin brushing and you'll start to see results.

Do It: Dry skin brush for about three minutes before your morning shower.

Floss: Flossing is that important. Seriously. When we floss, we reach places the toothbrush can't and so it is vital for getting rid of extra food bits that the bacteria in our mouths feed on, which leads to extra plaque buildup and nasty breath. When you don't floss, you're actually missing more than one-third of your tooth's surface. Imagine if every time you showered you didn't clean the same one-third of your body? And what if those body parts were the deep, dark ones where bacteria and grime could make a home. Barftown! Within twenty-four to thirty-six hours, plaque hardens into tough stuff, which the professionals call tartar.

Do It: It is recommended to floss at least once a day, but we should probably floss as many times as we eat.

Focus on the Exhale: In two-three-four, out two-three-four. And repeat. That is how our breath goes. When we get focused on a task, when we get stressed, or when we sit hunched over our keyboard, dinner plate, or steering wheel, we breathe very shallowly. This shallow breathing moves us deeper into a stressed, fight-or-flight, adrenaline-fueled state. Further, hunching over compresses our chest, making it tougher to breathe deeply and also puts our body into the posture of depression and low energy. As soon as we sit up straight and pull our shoulders back, whether standing or sitting, our energy is immediately boosted. Similarly, taking a few very deep, full breaths, filling the lungs to their maximum capacity and slowly exhaling, will boost our energy and calm our mood. Easy as that.

Do It: Make a conscious effort to start and end each day with a few massive deep breaths, maintaining a steady focus on the exhale. When in states of

2

3

stress, work on making the exhale move out two or three times slower than your deep inhale. This slow exhale technique can also work wonders to quiet your mind chatter and help you sleep.

4

Sit Still: While we're on the topic of deep breathing, how is that brain spin of yours? Often stress leaves our body feeling a lot like it did coming in, which can make sitting in meditation a seemingly stressful and anxiety-ridden activity. Do it anyway. It gets easier. Stress is not attractive, so we need to take on practices that help us loosen it up and shake it out. Happy and relaxed is where we want to be. Never feel guilty for doing absolutely nothing because you work hard for that nothing and in doing nothing – well, that is where the magic happens. If stopping the "doings" cold turkey is too much, try lying on your back, holding your knees in, and rolling from side to side just because it feels nice; take a hot bath without books, phones, or computers (lovers are allowed); go for a walk without a destination; or drink a cup of tea in silence and appreciate how good it makes you feel. Just be a little still. This stillness will make a whole lot of space for creativity to pour into your life. Remember that the days where you think you are too busy to be still are the days that you need it the most.

Do It: You can combine this with the deep breathing if you like, but find some time every day to be a little still and focus inward – not on your thoughts but on the stillness and the breath. Focus on the exhale.

5

The Power of Pooping: There is really nothing quite like a good poop to start your day off right. I'm serious. There are a few key things that need to be in place in order to ensure a good, healthy morning elimination. Fiber and water are part of the equation, but timing and rhythm are another. In order to have a proper poop, you need to allow time for it to happen. Set ten minutes aside every morning to visit the "home office." Take some reading materials with you and just relax. The body works in cycles and patterns and setting up this time as part of your routine will help make it happen. In case you're curious, a proper poop is going to be large, full, and well-formed, likely with a bit of an S-curve to it. It should plop gently, glide through the water, and shouldn't require too much wiping. Too much info? I'm not looking for a photo report.

Just start paying attention and making it happen. With a good poop in the morning, you'll have more energy through the day, feel (and be!) physically lighter, and over time, you'll notice improvements in your digestive health as well as in your physical appearance, with a flatter belly and clearer skin.

Do It: Make your daily poop happen. Start by making time for it. Head in to the sanctuary with a good book every day at the same time. Let your body know this is the time for action. Add some dietary adjustments such as more fiber and water, maybe a good probiotic supplement, and take on some relaxation activities in the morning such as walking or stretching. Make a morning poop part of your morning routine, just like brushing your teeth and bathing – all part of getting fresh and ready for the day.

Make a Sock Puppet . . . or Paint a Picture: What's your favorite hobby? Have you forgotten? As we near the end of UnDiet, I am going to wish upon the stars that your new fave hobby might be playing in the kitchen while having your daily exercise dance party. As we get older, we forget about the importance of play. We no longer have tap-dance classes, arts-and-crafts camp, or piano lessons to remind us of that little creative streak deep down inside. Get in touch with it, grab hold, make time, and let it come out to play. Creativity helps people stay healthy.[1] If you're not the type to take on a craft project at home, perhaps there's a way to take on a creative project at work, whether it be planning a staff event or creating an UnDiet Task Force.

Do It: Take part in some creative task every day. This can be anything from journaling to knitting to throwing a dance party and making up new moves. Let yourself loosen the goosen, be a little silly, and create something without giving thought to any desired outcome.

6

Change Your Routine with Purpose: Our brains are going to kick and scream at us as soon as we propose a shake-up of the usual, which is why changing habits is so tough. The little part of the brain called the amygdala registers a stress response when we take on big shifts. It can therefore be delightfully helpful to make a few itty-bitty changes every day to help lighten the stress load of the big ones. This is why gradual modifications tend to stick best. Find little things in your everyday life that you can switch around. Maybe rearrange

7

photos on your fireplace mantel, take a different route to work, or shop the supermarket from the opposite way you normally do. It's amazing what we may notice, experience, and discover when we change our vantage point.

Do It: Make some changes. Any changes will do. Find at least one little thing every day that you can change up, change around, or do differently and see how it feels, what may come of it, or just practice getting a little comfortable with the uncomfortable.

8 **Stretch. Move. Bounce:** A full workout isn't always needed or possible, but that's not to say that you are then better off doing nothing at all. There is massive benefit to walking for just twenty minutes every day, doing twenty minutes of sun salutations at home, or kicking off your shoes and jumping on the bed (though watch out for lights and ceiling fans). A little movement every day will increase your metabolic rate, calm your mind, boost your circulation and just make you feel good all over.

Do It: Commit to a little bit of moving for the sake of moving every day. Walking up and down the grocery aisle doesn't count. Take twenty minutes in the morning to stretch and breathe, get off one stop early on your way to work, or take off all your clothes (or not) and dance till you can't dance no more. Just move.

get the stories
behind the photos
http://bit.ly/UnDiet

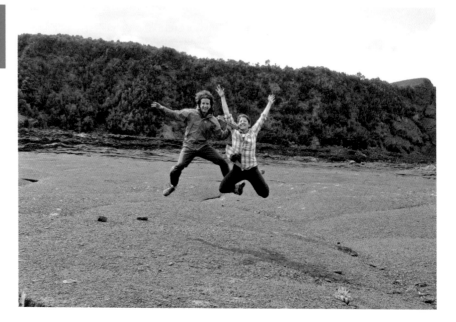

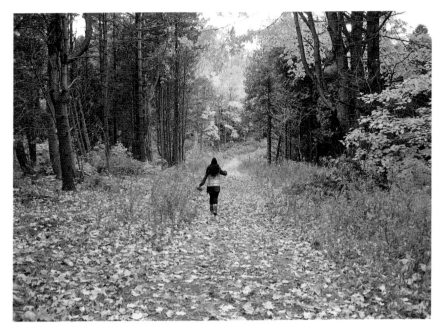

Surround Yourself with Beauty: Personally, when I am outdoors, preferably in a location where I can't hear cars or see city lights, I consider it a pretty beautiful place to be. You have to determine what brings joy to your eyes, your nose, your feet and all the other senses we need to stimulate regularly, and make it happen. Clutter, typically, is a pretty tough place to hang out in. Creating a chillaxing environment that you find appealing to all your senses will bring forth a calm, quiet peace like no other. Given that our low-impact living has done away with the consumption of disposables, we're done with spending lots of money on cheap, poor-quality stuff that only clutters the space. The new strategy is one of selectivity, where we save up until we can afford a few good-quality items that really make us happy. Quality (and beauty) over quantity.

Do It: Can you get rid of something every day? Probably not. Can you stop buying stuff every day? Totally! Keep things tidy, dump the clutter that spoils your environment; and make every effort to create a space that feels great to be in.

Laugh. Really Hard: I have saved the best for last. My day just isn't complete unless, at some point, I've had a really solid, hearty laugh. If tears come, I can't catch my breath and have to run off to the loo to tinkle in a

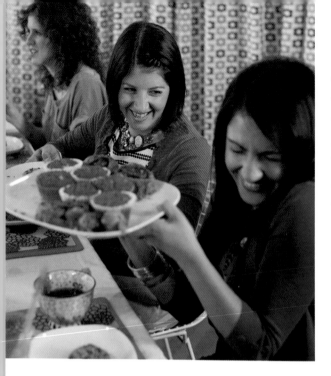

quick sprint, then it is a laugh worth laughing. Laughter truly is the very best medicine. A good laugh can help to relieve physical tension, decrease stress hormones, and increase immune cells and infection-fighting antibodies. A good old chuckle triggers the release of endorphins, the body's natural feel-good chemicals that promote feelings of well-being and affect us on a cellular level. This simple act stimulates key immune system cells, specifically natural killer cells, the white blood cells that helps destroy cancerous tumors.

Do It: Laugh at the ridiculousness of seriousness once, maybe twice a day. There is humor in most things and if we can spend a little time looking for it, well, we just might find a laugh in there.

THE LAST LITTLE PIECES OF THE PUZZLE: YOU!

Way back long ago at the start of this journey, we took it upon ourselves to question some rather weighty paradigms that have, quite literally, been weighing us down for some time.

It has been drilled into us that all great results require some dramatic and often aggressive intervention. We all want to be that six-week makeover story. What happens, though, after another six weeks have passed? All too often it is an easy-come, easy-go scenario. The joy of fitting into your high-school prom dress only lasts so long when you're completely starving and your nervous system is shot from working out too hard without eating fully powered, real whole food.

What do we do? We seek the pill. And the modern medical approach all too often reinforces this. First come meds, and then come supplements, which are still pills in which we put a lot of faith. The next recommendation is usually of some type of dietary limitation. The fourth component is lifestyle where we are told to sleep and exercise more. Attitude becomes the last thing we consider addressing. Rather than dig deep on down to address the baggage we drag around that puts wrinkles in even our cutest ensemble, we are sent off to a shrink and put on meds to numb the attitude problem into submission. We get turned into sheeple, believing we need to follow the herd.

Here's the catch: we can never achieve optimal health with just diet and the right supplements. We can get all up in arms about drinking the best water, taking the best digestive enzymes, the best probiotics, and eating the best of the best biodynamic organic spinach, but when we're miserable, no amount of salad will heal our woes. The specifics around diet are part of the super health equation.

You have to love what you see when you look in the mirror, but you have to love even more what you feel when you close your eyes, sit quiet, and follow your breath. That is the place where ultimate health, happiness, and beauty come from.

No vibrant lifestyle program would be full and complete without a few key tricks and tips to ensure we continue along the health-building side of the playing field. Of all the goodness I love to share, these strategies to ensure we stay within the sunshiny bits of our mind, only allowing a few poor-little-me moments to poke around on a rare occasion, are what truly keep us keeping on.

TRY THE SILVER LINING ON FOR SIZE

We chatted, you and I, not long ago about that whole idea of a glass being half-empty or half-full and looking for the one that overflows. What about that pesky habit we have of failing to notice what is contained inside that glass and instead focusing on the small crack in the side? This can and should be changed.

Sure, people and jobs may irk the irks right out of you. Perhaps these times give you the opportunity to step away and see what there is that you love. There is a fine balance here between looking for the silver lining, opening up to focus on the good, and making excuses or allowing ourselves to continue to suffer because of the bad. You know what I'm saying? Your job can legitimately blow, and you may have good reason for your complaining about it – for a short time. The same goes with the loverly lover with whom you share your life. Our emotions and circumstances will naturally flow in waves with ups and downs. That's okay. Honesty has to come in at some point when we ask ourselves if, when we look at the big picture, we are feeling good or bad, happy or sad, full of joy or despair.

Vibrant health is infinite, when we are feeling fulfilled, at peace, and happy. At the same time, this can ultimately be limited and impaired by the way we perceive and process the circumstances of our lives. In other words, our emotional misery will put a cap on how physically well we can be.

Stress will come and go as a natural part of life, but we need to find ways to manage and deal with it. At the end of the day, I can only stand to listen to you complain about your mean partner, nasty boss, or messed up digestion for so long if you continually have excuses to not change anything. Sleep and exercise will help to boost the mood, but if you are miserable all day long at work and then dread going home 'cause you can't stand the person waiting for you, there is a pretty good chance your health goals will remain just out of reach.

What often happens is that things get rough in one bit of our lives and we start to transfer it to all the others. My fair lady friends, we are known for many things but compartmentalizing our emotions is not one of them. There are, however, easy tools and exercises that can be tried and tested to help us fall in love with each and every single day.

A massive change in your life may not be the answer. All that may be needed is a minor switch in how you think about things – and this could have massive power. Doing the same thing over and over and expecting different results, I do believe, is the definition of insanity. If what you're doing isn't working for you, it's time to shake it up. In order to fall in love every day and find that silver lining, we may need to make huge leaps and bounds that take heroic shows of bravery. The huge leap could be as massive as quitting your job and moving to the Caribbean to sell custom-made coconut husk bracelets on the beach (don't you dare steal my retirement plan), or talking out an issue with another person rather than shutting down and walking away. The shake up, however, could simply be in doing the same thing you do every day, but doing it differently.

The real act of bravery is simply in being true enough to yourself to respond to your inherent desire to be happy, and making your own happiness a priority. That is where your desired state of health is going to prosper.

ATTITUDE IS JUST ABOUT EVERYTHING

We have now fully embraced the ridiculous radness of clean, low-impact, health-supportive eating. For the most part, the lifestyle essentially takes care of itself and once we begin to feel amazing in our body, our mood naturally lifts to one of optimism, productivity, and hopefully a sense of calm from knowing that you, yes you, Little Miss Thang, are in full control of your health.

Instead of going from meds to supplements to diet to lifestyle to attitude – we flip this pattern upside down and shake it up. We use the great food we feed ourselves in partnership with some lifestyle changes, and a sense of fun and humor to motivate a healthier, more fulfilled, and nourished lifestyle. We have no choice but to address some of our attitude and mood stuff along the way. You didn't even notice, did you?

So what then is that final super important component? It's the simplest stuff of all, though often the toughest to heal and repair. Remember way back when we were talking about breaking habits and I suggested getting a group of people together who really and truly want to see us succeed? Sometimes, as we regain our health, suddenly the fog that has been covering our spectacles is lifted and we start seeing things clearly. We may begin to recognize a dissatisfaction with the limitations of our job, the impact of a challenging relationship, or perhaps how defeated we feel after being pushed too far by a trainer at the gym.

"Frustration and Love can't exist in the same place at the same time, so get real and start doing what you would rather be doing in life. Love your life. All of it. Even the heavy shit that happened to you when you were 8. All of it was and is perfect."
– Jason Mraz

As we begin to treat ourselves better, we begin to expect others to treat us better too. As we demand more from ourselves, strive for more, and are capable of more, we look to find outlets and resources to fully express our own personal amazingness. We want to be recognized for our full potential and encouraged to express it. Give yourself a pat on the back for that! When we raise that bar of how we think of and care for ourselves, that bar gets raised in all aspects of our lives.

The grand missing component of total health is our attitude. We can

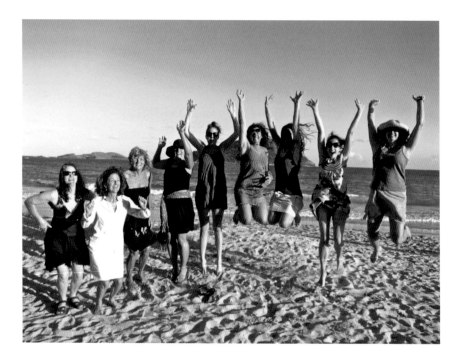

blame others all we want but ultimately our level of health and happiness is our own responsibility. It is about how much we love the job that we do all day, how much we exercise and move and enjoy it, how much deep rest and relaxation we get, how much we love and enjoy the company of those we have chosen to love and enjoy, and generally how happy we are. This small but mighty piece of the health puzzle is the greatest determinant of super UnDiet success.

UNDIET LIVING

UnDiet for Abundance Mantra

Health, happiness, joy, and calm are here and now.

Make Love in the Kitchen

❋ Scrap the to-do list once in a while to make time for yourself.

❋ Nothing that important happens after 10:00 p.m. Go to sleep!

❋ Take on the little things to see the big results.

❋ Change your mind and see what unfolds.

TRANSITIONAL TIPS AND TRICKS TO MAKE IT HAPPEN

❋ Make time to move.

Exercise is a cumulative thing, so make the time every day to take on activities you love, even if just a little bit. Twenty minutes of movement a day is a non-negotiable. Come on, now, shake it!

❋ Track the goodness.

Pay attention every day to the goodness, the things that bring a smile to your face, make you feel good, or what you have done to bring happiness to another. Journal it or just jot it down quickly. Marinade in those moments of joy as you drift off to sleep and watch your life transform.

❋ Sit and be still.

Find the time every day to bring a little stillness and quiet into your life and into your mind. The abundance that will flow from these quiet moments is beyond awesometown.

❋ Sleep deep.

Create your sleep sanctuary, establish your sleep routine, and put it into effect. Generally we need eight hours of sleep a night to maintain health. We're going to need a few extra Zs to regain our health.

❋ Take it all in.

It is a luxury that we can choose our lifestyle. Though we can't always dictate or own big changes, we can always choose the little things – namely how we respond to what life throws our way. Find the silver lining as best you can, wrap yourself up in it, and have a good laugh at it all.

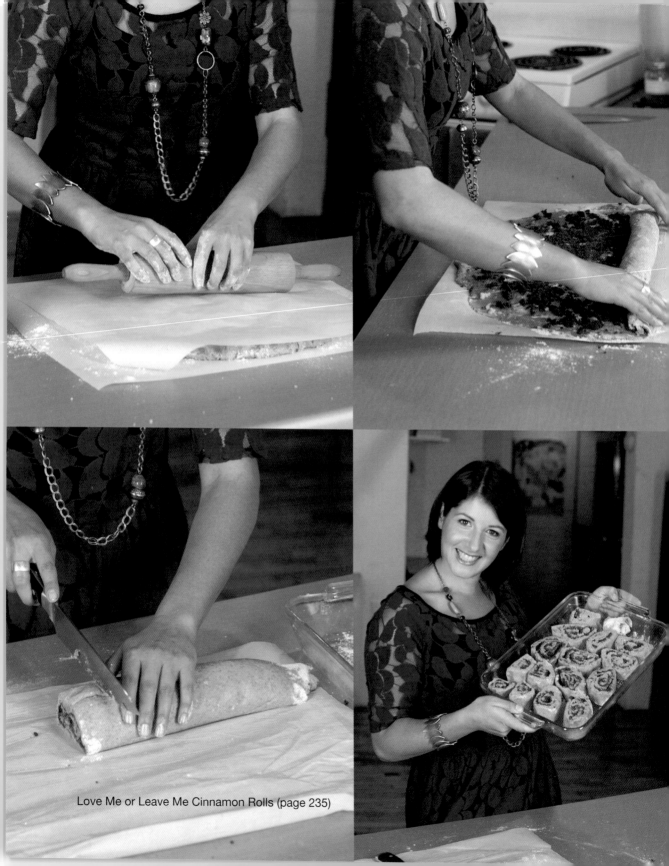

Love Me or Leave Me Cinnamon Rolls (page 235)

Love Me or Leave Me Cinnamon Rolls

Makes: about 12 rolls

DOUGH

DRY INGREDIENTS

2 cups	brown rice flour	500 mL
1 cup	buckwheat flour	250 mL
1 cup	arrowroot starch	250 mL
1 tbsp	baking powder	15 mL
1 tsp	baking soda	5 mL
1 tsp	sea salt	5 mL
1 tsp	cinnamon	5 mL

WET INGREDIENTS

1 cup	butternut squash or sweet potato, steamed	250 mL
1 cup	applesauce	250 mL
¼ cup	maple syrup	50 mL
2 tbsp	raw honey	30 mL
½ cup	coconut oil	125 mL
2 tsp	vanilla extract	10 mL

FILLING

½ cup	coconut sugar, or Sucanat, powdered in coffee grinder	125 mL
¼ cup	raw cocoa powder (optional)	50 mL
¼ cup	cinnamon	50 mL
	pinch of clove	
	pinch of nutmeg	
	pinch of sea salt	
⅓ cup	coconut oil, softened to the consistency of room temperature butter	75 mL

DOUGH DIRECTIONS

- Preheat oven to 350°F (180°C).
- Grease an 11- x 9-inch glass baking dish and dust with brown rice flour. Set aside.
- In a large bowl, mix dry ingredients.
- Place wet ingredients in the food processor, and mix until smooth. Wipe down the sides of the bowl with a spatula as needed.
- Add the wet ingredients to the dry, and mix, scraping the sides of the bowl. If the dough is too sticky to roll, add a little more buckwheat flour.
- Place the dough between two pieces of parchment paper. If the dough is still too sticky, sprinkle with a little more buckwheat flour. (Too much flour will make the rolls dense and dry.)
- Use a rolling pin to form the dough into a rectangular shape.

FILLING DIRECTIONS

- In a small bowl, mix the sweetener, cocoa, cinnamon, clove, nutmeg, and sea salt.
- Spread coconut oil evenly over the dough, and sprinkle the powder mix generously over the entire surface of the dough rectangle.
- Grasp the edge of the parchment paper farthest from you and roll the dough inwards to create a long snake. Use the parchment to help roll.
- With a sharp knife, cut slices about 2–3 inches (5–8 cm) thick, and place them close together in the glass baking dish. The closer they are packed, the moister the rolls will be.
- Bake for 20–30 minutes. Serve warm or allow to cool, and store airtight in the freezer for one month.

Life-Affirming Chili

Serves: 6

2 tbsp	extra virgin olive oil	30 mL
1	onion, coarsely chopped	1
1 tbsp	ginger root, grated	15 mL
2	garlic cloves, minced	2
2 tsp	turmeric	10 mL
2 tbsp	dried basil	30 mL
2 tbsp	dried oregano	30 mL
1 tsp	dried thyme	5 mL
15 oz	can organic kidney beans	425 g
15 oz	can organic white or navy beans	425 g
3	carrots, coarsely chopped	3
2	stalks of celery, coarsely chopped	2
2	medium tomatoes, seeded and coarsely chopped	2
1 tbsp	raw honey	15 mL
2 cups	water (add more as needed, depending on desired consistency)	500 mL
	pinch each of cinnamon, all spice, nutmeg	
	sea salt and cayenne to taste	

DIRECTIONS

- Heat the olive oil in a large saucepan. Add the onions and sauté until translucent, about 5 minutes. Add the ginger and garlic and cook for another 2 minutes.

- Add spices and stir until thoroughly mixed together and slightly aromatic. Stir in beans, carrots, celery, tomatoes, and honey, then gradually add water to avoid making it too soupy.

- Cover and let simmer for 45 minutes. If the chili is too watery, simmer uncovered while stirring occasionally for another 10–15 minutes.

- Add sea salt and cayenne to taste. Serve hot.

Chocolate Love
Almond Butter Cups

Serves: 12 almond butter cups in a muffin tin, or 24 in candy molds

CHOCOLATE

⅓ cup	raw cocoa powder	75 mL
¼ cup	coconut oil	50 mL
¼ cup	raw cocoa butter	50 mL
2 tbsp	raw honey	30 mL

Note: You can replace raw cocoa powder and raw cocoa butter with 1 bar (¾ cup / 175 mL) baker's chocolate.

FILLING

⅓ cup	almond butter	75 mL
1 tbsp	dried shredded coconut, ground further in a coffee grinder	15 mL
1 tbsp	raw honey	15 mL
1 tsp	arrowroot starch	5 mL
	pinch of sea salt	

DIRECTIONS

- Over low heat, melt together the cocoa powder, coconut oil, cocoa butter, and raw honey.
- Pour a small amount of chocolate into each well of the muffin tin, enough to cover the bottom. Place in freezer for 10 minutes or until solid.
- Blend the filling ingredients in a small bowl. Set aside.
- Remove chocolate from freezer, form small patties of the filling mixture, and gently place over the chocolate in the muffin tin, leaving room all the way around to fill in with chocolate.
- Reheat the chocolate mix, if needed, then spoon chocolate into each muffin cup until filling is completely covered, and return muffin tin to freezer for about 30–40 minutes to allow chocolate to set.
- Serve chilled.

Apple-Cinnamon Bedtime Snack

1	apple, sliced thinly or cut in ½-inch (1-cm) cubes	1
1 tsp	cinnamon	5 mL
1 tbsp	chopped pecans (optional)	15 mL
	maple syrup	

DIRECTIONS

- Steam the apple for about 8 minutes, or just until soft, then transfer to serving bowl, and toss with cinnamon and drizzle with maple syrup. Sprinkle with pecans if desired.
- Eat as is, top your favorite coconut ice cream, love with pancakes or French toast, or mix into your roasted vegetable.

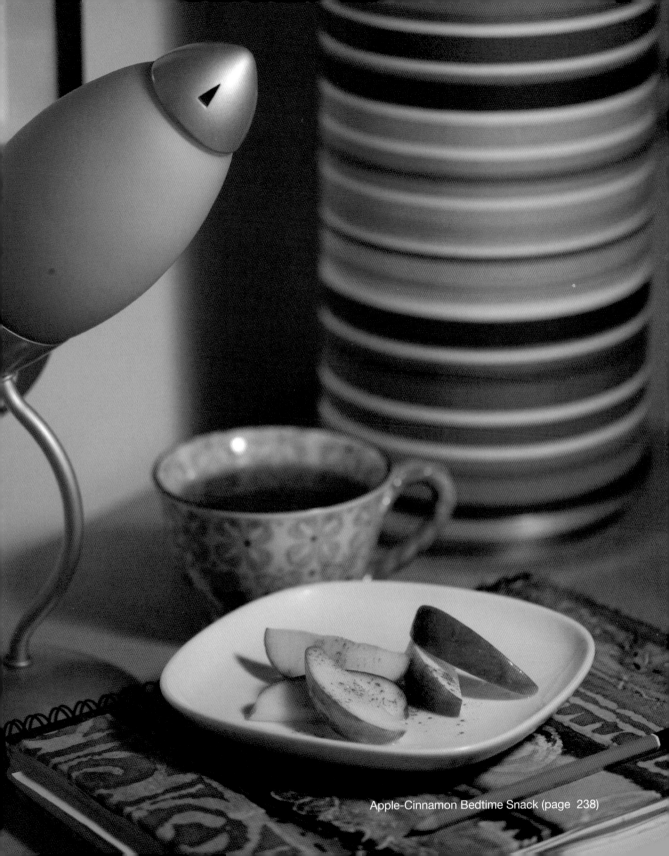

Apple-Cinnamon Bedtime Snack (page 238)

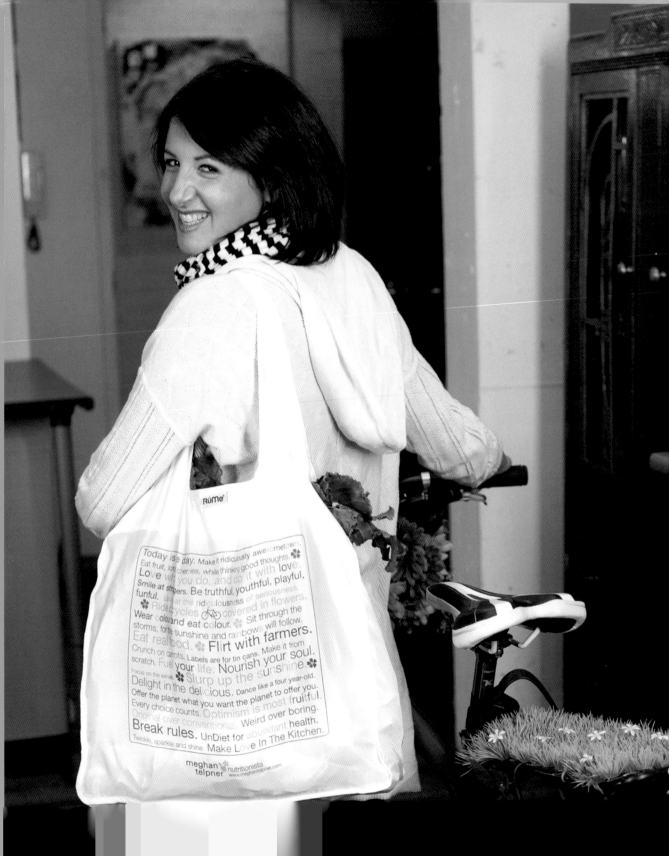

Today is the day. Make it ridiculously awesometown.
Eat fruit, lots cherries, while thinking good thoughts. ❀
Love what you do, and do it with love.
Smile at strangers. Be truthful, youthful, playful,
funful. Laugh at the ridiculousness of seriousness.
❀ Ride bicycles covered in flowers. ❀
Wear colour and eat colour. ❀ Sit through the
storms, for the sunshine and rainbows will follow.
Eat real food. ❀ Flirt with farmers.
Crunch on carrots. Labels are for tin cans. Make it from
scratch. Fuel your life. Nourish your soul.
Focus on the exhale. ❀ Slurp up the sunshine. ❀
Delight in the delicious. Dance like a four year-old.
Offer the planet what you want the planet to offer you.
Every choice counts. Optimism is most fruitful.
Original over conventional. Weird over boring.
Break rules. UnDiet for abundant health.
Twinkle, sparkle and shine. Make Love In The Kitchen.

meghan
telpner nutritionista
www.meghantelpner.com

And There You Have It

That wasn't so hard was it? You're thinking, *How on earth did I ever live my life up until now without knowing all this stuff and doing so many of these easy little things to improve my health?* Or maybe you're spinning this idea: *That Meghan. She is something else. Pretty kooky, but she sure made me think.*

All of those thoughts are exactly right. You, my UnDiet ambassador, just have to pick up where you can and take it as far as you can handle. You can dig that for sure. My only suggestion is that you continue on with these transitions, taking them on one or two at a time, and keep them up as best you can. If you find yourself too stressed by it all, consider these two things:

✿ **You are blessed to be stressed!** Recognize how lucky you are that your stress of the day is whether you have the time to go for a twenty minute walk, or that you are out of mason jars to pack your lunch, or whether to have blueberry pancakes for breakfast or a green smoothie. These are some sweet, lucky problems to have. For sure you are allowed to be stressed about the changes, but perspective is a magical tool for getting ourselves over ourselves.

✿ **Don't do it all!** That's an easy one, right? If too much too soon is just too much for you, then take it back a few steps. Do what you can, as you can do it. Make it maintainable and sustainable, pushing yourself every so often to your edge, but never feeling the need to go so far that you fall right off. We don't do cheat days around here. We do the best we can. That's it, that's all.

I am not letting you go just yet. There is still much goodness you best be using, referencing, and loving. I have put together a sweet little transition schedule for you and taken all the recipes from the book and tied them up into an awesome meal plan. The fun never stops in the kitchen.

Hip, hip, hooray for the UnDiet Revolution that is about to unfold. You are a revolutionary in this movement and you and I together – we're leading the way!

LET'S DO THIS:
YOUR 8-WEEK TRANSFORMATION!

As you went through the book, you learned a whole lot. Let this 8-Week Transformation be your guide.

WEEK 1

* Drink eight to ten glasses of water a day. About 2 quarts (2 liters) is preferred. (Page 42)
* Start your day with lemon and cayenne in 8–16 ounces (250–500 mL) of water. (Page 55)
* Replace at least one coffee or black tea with an herbal alternative. (Page 50)
* Add extra greens to your juices. (Page 49)
* Nix the ice from your drinks. (Page 42)

WEEK 2

* Go grocery shopping with a list. (Page 96)
* Challenge yourself to only buy package-free foods. (Page 174)
* Ask where your food comes from. (Page 64)

WEEK 3

* Create a menu for the week. (Page 92)
* Prep veggies when they're fresh. (Page 98)
* Brown bag your lunch a minimum of two to three days a week. (Page 105)

WEEK 4

* Fill your plate just once. (Page 122)
* Put down your fork down between bites and eat slowly. (Page 122)
* Set the table, with napkins and all. (Page 113)
* Make time in your schedule to eat – at least thirty minutes per day. (Page 123)
* Share a meal with friends, family, or co-workers. (Page 125)

WEEK 5

❋ Choose three goals and identify habits that are keeping you from achieving them. (Page 147)

❋ Eliminate refined sugar from your diet – choose whole, healthier sweetener options. (Page 154)

❋ Deal with your emotions – do not use food as a distraction. (Page 136)

❋ Catch you later, caffeine – ease yourself off slowly. (Page 145)

❋ Build a team that supports your goals. (Page 148)

WEEK 6

❋ Start storing food in glass instead of plastic. (Page 172)

❋ Make three of your favorite staples from scratch. (Page 177)

❋ Clean out the crap and donate gently used items to a local charity or thrift store. (Page 174)

WEEK 7

❋ Choose three days out of the week that you limit your makeup. (Page 199)

❋ Cut the products you use daily down to half. (Page 199)

❋ Choose non-toxic options for the products you use daily. (Page 199)

❋ Mix your own home-cleaning products. (Page 205)

❋ Use the cash you save to pamper yourself. (Page 207)

WEEK 8

❋ Make time to shake your booty. (Page 216)

❋ Marinade in the moments of joy in your day. (Page 231)

❋ Sit and be still. Find the time to meditate and reflect. (Page 224)

❋ Create your sleep sanctuary, establish your routine, and put it into effect. (Page 221)

❋ Find the silver lining as best you can, wrap yourself up in it, and have a good laugh at it all. (Page 229)

UNDIET MEAL PLAN

	DAY 1	DAY 2	DAY 3
Upon Waking	Lemon, Cayenne, and Water	Lemon, Cayenne, and Water	Lemon, Cayenne, and Water
Breakfast	Blue-Green Power Smoothie	Whole-Grain Porridge + Yogi Tea	Blueberry Pancakes + Yogi Tea
Snack	Sun-dried Tomato and Bean Hummus with mixed veggies	Pretty Me Latte	Herbed Quinoa Sesame Crackers topped with sliced tomatoes and cucumber
Lunch	Lemon Lentil Vegetable Soup and Herbed Quinoa Sesame Crackers	Cran-Apple Green Salad with Honey-Cider Dressing	One-Pot Stir-Fry over mixed greens
Snack	Herbal Mocha Latte	Spiced Apple-Carrot Muffin	Apple-Cinnamon Bedtime Snack
Dinner	One-Pot Stir-Fry	Bean and Vegetable Burger with steamed vegetables	Orange Zest–Infused Stew on quinoa

DAY 4	DAY 5	DAY 6	DAY 7
Lemon, Cayenne, and Water	Lemon, Cayenne, and Water	Lemon, Cayenne, and Water	Lemon, Cayenne, and Water
Blue-Green Power Smoothie	My Favorite Granola with Freshly Blended Nut/Seed Milk and fresh fruit	Morning Green Juice Shazaam	Love Me Or Leave Me Cinnamon Rolls
Cucumber slices with Curried Caper Tahini Sauce	Apple-Cinnamon Bedtime Snack	Yogi Tea with 2 tsp coconut oil stirred in	Almond Power Cookies
Bean and Vegetable Burger and Quinoa Tabbouleh	Homemade Vegetable Stock with brown rice and Herbed Quinoa Sesame Crackers	Lemon Lentil Vegetable Soup and cucumber slices with Curried Caper Tahini Sauce	Life-Affirming Chili
Almond Power Cookies	Banana Chocolate Soft Serve	My Favorite Granola with Freshly Blended Nut/ Seed Milk	Cucumber slices with Curried Caper Tahini Sauce
Life-Affirming Chili and mixed greens with Honey-Cider Dressing	Meghan's No-Longer-Secret Tomato Sauce with chickpeas over buckwheat soba noodles	Booyizzle White Bean Green Curry	Veggie Rice Wraps with Almond Dipping Sauce

ACKNOWLEDGEMENTS

Today is the day. Together, let's make it ridiculously awesometown. It is only ever as awesome as those I share it with, those who inspire me, and those who help me to bring my brightest and biggest dreams into real life. If getting sick was the worst thing that ever happened to me, finding my way to health has been the greatest blessing.

My first pom-pom-filled thank you is for my peeps – my loyal readers, class guests, and clients, who cheer me on when I'm going strong and cheer me up on the storm-cloud days. None of this would have happened if you hadn't picked up what I've been putting down.

I wouldn't be able to teach the way I do without having the guidance that I have had. I am forever indebted to my greatest teachers: Bryan Kest, who taught me the value of looking within; Thom Knoles, who showed me a way to stop tearing down the brick wall to find the open door; and Ping and Dr. Ha for accelerating the healing of my body, being my first teachers of health and my closest family while I was in LA. Collectively, you guided me along on this healing journey and let me soar to find my own space within it.

Bhavna Chauhan, you discovered me! The day you left me a voice mail that had me cartwheeling, human pyramiding, and doing pop-a-wheelies until I could compose myself enough to call you back is the day that changed the game I was playing. You got me, ate what I cooked for you (and loved it), heard my voice, and invited me to share it – made-up words and all. You have as much enthusiasm for this project as I do, and that is hard to match. Ms. B, I love your edits, but you can keep your 142 Post-it notes. The team at McClelland & Stewart – thank you! I never knew "Meghan" could be an adjective until a four-day photo shoot that left us asking whether shots were "Meghan enough." Catherine Farquharson, you are officially the documen-tographer of my life. My friend first, and a partner on this project second; I want to see the world through your lens. It's pretty in there.

Thank you, Maeve Gallagher, my right-hand woman. You preserved my sanity. Sondi Bruner, you saved me from drowning in the aforementioned 142 Post-it notes. Much thanks to Joanne Hall and Chef Kristin Rugg Dovbniak for being the kitchen fairies during the hectic photo shoot. Lisa Borden, thank you doesn't cut it. You are my mentor, coach, ultimate bossy pants, and friend. You challenge me, believe in me, and, more than anything, get me.

Love and so much appreciation to my long-time friends for sticking around when I was too sick to come out and play, and accepting the version of me that emerged, loving me all the same. Most of all, thank you to my family. My mom Patsy and dad Ron, my brother Michael, sis-in-law Carly, and sweet Mia Jean – without you I wouldn't have ridiculous anecdotes to share, and just might start taking all of this too seriously. The quirkiness of our family is my normal and for that I am grateful. Thank you for making meals that play by the UnDiet rules; the greatest source of support is that you are living this lifestyle right along with me. Mom and Dad, thank you a gabillion times over. You gave me the freedom to choose my path, supported me during my struggles, and celebrated the sweetness of the successes. Every experience I have had in my life that was worth having is because of you.

I will forever be in wonder for the joy that has continued to flow into my life since I found this path. Through my passion for health, I found my greatest teacher, bestest friend, professional colleague, fellow activist, travel partner, soul mate, and husband Josh Gitalis. From you I have learned more than I can even begin to quantify. You once told me that if I wished hard enough for unicorns, they would start to show up at my door. This just might be true as having you by my side is as sure a sign as any that all of my dreams do come true. With all my heart, we will "here and now" forever together, continuing toward the path of true and optimal health for ourselves and always assist those who seek our guidance.

And now, collectively, let's twinkle, sparkle and shine, make love in the kitchen, and UnDiet our way to the life of our dreams.

NOTES

Chapter 1

[1] Canadian Cancer Research Alliance. Cancer Research Investment in Canada, 2008: The Canadian Cancer Research Alliance's Survey of Government and Voluntary Sector Investment in Cancer Research in 2008, (Toronto: CCRA, 2011). [September 29, 2011] http://www.ccra-acrc.ca/PDF%20Files/Annual_2008_EN.pdf.

[2] "Cancer Research Funding," National Cancer Institute. [September 29, 2011] http://www.cancer.gov/cancertopics/factsheet/NCI/research-funding.

[3] Centers for Disease Control and Prevention, "Overweight and Obesity," last modified February 27, 2012, [October 3rd, 2011], http://www.cdc.gov/obesity/data/trends.html.

[4] "Metabolic & Bariatric Surgery Fact Sheet." American Society for Metabolic & Bariatric Surgery. Metabolic & Bariatric Surgery Fact Sheet. Revised: June 2010.

[5] "Top 200 Drugs for 2010 by sales, " Pharmaceutical Sales 2010 Access, April 8, 2012 http://www.drugs.com/top200.html.

[6] Nicolas Bakalar, "Prescription Drug Use Soared in Past Decade," New York Times, [October 3, 2010] http://www.nytimes.com/2010/10/19/health/research/19stats.html.

[7] Robert Longley, "Almost Half of Americans Take at Least One Prescription Drug," About.com U.S. Government Info, [September 29, 2011] http://usgovinfo.about.com/od/healthcare/a/usmedicated.htm.

[8] Ibid.

[9] Drew Falkenstein, "E. coli 0157:57 in Ground Beef . . . Yet Again," Food Poison Journal, November 3, 2009, [October 14, 2011] http://www.foodpoisonjournal.com/food-borne-illness-outbreaks/e-coli-o157h7-in-ground-beef-yet-again/.

Chapter 2

[1] Earl S. Ford, Wayne H. Gyles, and William H. Dietz, "Prevalence of the Metabolic Syndrome Among U.S. Adults," Journal of American Medical Association, October 16, 2007. [October 14th, 2011] http://www.phys.mcw.edu/documents/paper6prevalenceofmetabolicsyndrome.pdf.

[2] Natalie D. Riediger and Ian Clara, "Prevalence of Metabolic Syndrome in the Canadian Adult Population," Canadian Medical Association Journal, 183 (15) October 18, 2011 (first published September 12, 2011). [October 26, 2011] http://www.cmaj.ca/content/183/15/E1127.full.

[3] Gina Kolata, "Vitamins: More May Be Too Many," *New York Times*, April 29, 2003 [October 14th, 2011] http://www.nytimes.com/2003/04/29/science/vitamins-more-may-be-too-many.html?pagewanted=all&src=pm.

[4] Statistics Canada, *Canadian Health Measures Survey*, January 13, 2010. [October 26, 2011] http://www.statcan.gc.ca/daily-quotidien/100113/dq100113a-eng.htm.

[5] "U.S. Obesity Trends," Centers for Disease Control and Prevention. [November 7, 2011] http://www.cdc.gov/obesity/data/trends.html.

Chapter 3

[1] Travis A. Smith, Biing-Hwan Lin, and Jong-Ying Lee, Taxing Caloric Sweetened Beverages: *Potential Effects on Beverage Consumption, Calorie Intake, and Obesity*, ERR-100, U.S. Department of Agriculture, Economic Research Service, July 2010. (Google eBook) DIANE Publishing, 2010.

[2] "Your Best Guide To Juicing Fruits and Vegetable," *The Juicing Book*. [April, 9, 2012] http://www.juicingbook.com/vegetables.

[3] World's Healthiest Foods, [April 8, 2012] http://www.whfoods.com.

[4] American Botanical Council, [April 8, 2012] http://cms.herbalgram.org/commissione/HerbIndex/approvedherbs.html.

Chapter 4

[1] "A Role for Sweet Taste: Calorie Predictive Relations in Energy Regulation by Rats," Susan E. Swithers, PhD and Terry L. Davidson, PhD, Purdue University; *Behavioral Neuroscience*, Vol. 122, No. 1.

[2] International Food Information Council Foundation and U.S. Food and Drug Administration, Food Ingredients and Colors, November 2004, revised April 2010, [November 3rd, 2011] http://www.fda.gov/Food/FoodIngredientsPackaging/ucm094211.htm.

[3] Altmedangel, "Top 20 Food Additives to Avoid" [November 3rd, 2011], http://altmed-angel.com/additive.htm.

[4] "Chemical Index," Environmental Working Group [April 9, 2012] http://www.ewg.org/chemindex.

[5] "All Ecolabels," EcolabelIndex.com [November 5th, 2011] http://www.ecolabelindex.com/ecolabels/.

[6] Mitch Lipka, "What Do Your Food Labels Really Mean, 'Free Range', 'Natural', 'Non-Toxic' and Other Myths" *Daily Finance*, June 7, 2010 [November 13th, 2011] http://www.dailyfinance.com/2010/05/07/what-do-your-food-labels-really-mean-free-range-natural/.

Chapter 5

[1] "Facebook Users Average 7 Hrs a Month in January as Digital Universe Expands," Nielson Wire (blog) Nielson.com, February 19, 2010. [November 19, 2011] http://blog.nielsen.com/nielsenwire/online_mobile/facebook-users-average-7-hrs-a-month-in-january-as-digital-universe-expands/.

Chapter 6

1. The National Center on Addiction and Substance Abuse at Columbia University, The Importance of Family Dinners VII, (New York: The National Center on Addiction and Substance Abuse at Columbia University, 2011). [December 2, 2011] http://www.casacolumbia.org/download.aspx?path=/UploadedFiles/b25fhksc.pdf.

2. Nancy Gibbs, "The Magic of the Family Meal," Time, June 4, 2006. [December 2, 2011] http://www.time.com/time/magazine/article/0,9171,1200760-2,00.html.

3. Ibid.

4. Ibid.

5. "Global and Regional food consumption patterns and trends," Food and Agriculture Organization of the United Nations, FAO Corporate Document Repository. April 4, 2012. http://www.fao.org/DOCREP/005/AC911E/ac911e05.htm.

Chapter 7

1. Magalie Lenoir, Fuschia Serre. Lauriane Cantin, Serge H. Ahmed, "Intense Sweetness Surpasses Cocaine Reward," PLoS ONE 2 (8). [November 20th, 2011] http://www.plosone.org/article/info:doi/10.1371/journal.pone.0000698.

2. Ibid.

3. "Sugar Can Be Addictive," Physorg.com, December 10, 2010. [November 16, 2011] http://www.physorg.com/news148116045.html.

4. Michael R. Eades, "A Spoonful of Sugar," The Blog of Michael R. Eades, M.D., http://www.proteinpower.com/drmike/sugar-and-sweeteners/a-spoonful-of-sugar/.

5. Gabriel Cousens, "Diabetic Cure," Natural News TV Interview, NaturalNewsUniversity.com. [April 8, 2012] http://tv.naturalnews.com/v.asp?v=16CFAC0ADF7F04C04B11D6E9DC098BCF. Gabriel Cousens interview with Mike Adams. [May, 2010] http://www.naturalnews.com/podcasts/Interview-Dr-Gabriel-Cousens.mp3.

Chapter 8

1. Mathis Wackernagel and William Rees, Our Ecological Footprint: Reducing Human Impact on the Earth (Gabriola, Island, B.C.: New Society, 1996) [Page 15]; and "U.S.A. is the country with the largest per capita footprint in the world – a footprint of 9.57 hectares. If everyone on the planet was to live like an average American, we would need 5 planets, or our current planet's biocapacity could only support about 1.2 billion people," from Much Ado About Nothing, October 11, 2006. [11/09/07] http://www.buynothing.biz/blog/index.php?itemid=13.

2. OECD Environmental Data Compendium, "Municipal Waste Generation (Most Recent) By country," Nationmaster.com, 2002. http://www.nationmaster.com/graph/env_mun_was_gen-environment-municipal-waste-generation.

3. "Basic Information about Food Waste," U.S. Environmental Protection Agency last updated February 8, 2012. http://www.epa.gov/osw/conserve/materials/organics/food/fd-basic.htm.

4. Martin Gooch, Abdel Felfel, and Nicole Marenek, Food Waste in Canada, (Guelph: Value Chain Management Centre, 2010), [pg. 2]. http://www.valuechains.ca/documents/Food%20Waste%20in%20Canada%2020120910.pdf.

5. "What a Waste: The Food We Throw Away," World Vision Canada. November 12, 2011] http://www.worldvision.ca/Education-and-Justice/advocacy-in-action/Pages/what-a-waste-the-food-we-throw-away.aspx.

6. "Basic Information about Food Waste," U.S. Environmental Protection Agency. [November 12, 2011] http://www.epa.gov/osw/conserve/materials/organics/food/fd-basic.htm.

7. Timothy W. Jones, "Using Contemporary Archaeology, and Applied Anthropology to Understand Food Loss in the American Food System," Bureau of Applied Research in Anthropology University of Arizona, Report to the United States Department of Agriculture, Economic Research Service, 2004.

8. Ibid.

9. Eye on Earth, "New Bans on Plastic Bags May Help Protect Marine Life," Worldwatch Institute.org, http://www.worldwatch.org/node/5565.

10. "Adverse Health Effects of Plastics," Ecology Center. [November 12, 2011] http://www.ecologycenter.org/factsheets/plastichealtheffects.html.

11. "The Disappearing Male," CBC Doc Zone, November 7th, 2008.

12. U.S. Food and Drug Administration, Update on Bisphenol A for Use in Food Contact Applications, January 2010. [November 26, 2011] http://www.fda.gov/newsevents/publichealthfocus/ucm064437.htm.

13. "Common Cancer Types," National Cancer Institute, November12, 2011. http://www.cancer.gov/cancertopics/types/commoncancers.

14. http://www.cleanair.org/Waste/wasteFacts.html. Wills, A. (June 21, 2010), *Recycling To-Go Plastics*. [June 2010] http://earth911.com/news/2010/06/21/recycling-to-go-plastics/.

15. Sadie B. Barr, and Jonathan C. Wright, "Postprandial Energy Expenditure in Whole-Food and Processed-Food Meals: Implications for Daily Energy Expenditure," Food and Nutrition Research, (July 2, 2010). [November 5, 2011] http://www.ncbi.nlm.nih.gov/pmc/articles/PMC2897733/.

16. Betsy Hornick and Eric Yarnell, "Health Benefits of Seeds," TLC Cooking. [November 20, 2011] http://recipes.howstuffworks.com/health-benefits-of-seeds-ga.htm.

Chapter 9

1. Jane Houlihan "Why This Matters, Cosmetics and Your Health," Environmental Working Group. [February 9, 2012] http://www.ewg.org/skindeep/2011/04/13/why-this-matters/.

2. "TSCA Enforcement Programs and Initiatives," U.S. Environmental Protection Agency, May 18, 2010. [February 9, 2012] http://www.epa.gov/compliance/civil/tsca/tscaenfprog.html.

3. "Table 1: Frank Carcinogens," Cancer Prevention Coalition. [November 30th, 2011] http://preventcancer.com/consumers/cosmetics/documents/Table1_FrankCarc_forweb_jun189.pdf

4. Paul H. McCay, Alain A. Ocampo-Sosa, and Gerard T. A. Fleming, "Effect of Subinhibitory Concentrations of Benzalkonium Chloride on the Competitiveness of Pseudomonas Aeruginosa Grown in Continuous Culture," *Microbiology*, 156 (1) (online October 8, 2009; print January 2010): 30–38. http://mic.sgmjournals.org/content/156/1/30.abstract.

5. Joseph Mercola, "Shocking Update – Sunshine Can Actually Decrease Your Vitamin D

Levels," Mercola.com, May 12 2009. http://articles.mercola.com/sites/articles/archive/2009/05/12/shocking-update-sunshine-can-actually-decrease-your-vitamin-d-levels.aspx.

Chapter 10

[1] John Mirowsky and Catherine E. Ross "Creative Work and Health," *Journal of Health and Social Behavior*, 48 (4) (December 2007): 385–403. [December 14, 2011] http://hsb.sagepub.com/content/48/4/385.abstract.

INDEX

RECIPE INDEX